MW00465443

COSMO'S SEXY SUTRA

COSMO'S SEXY SUTRA

101 EPIC SEX POSITIONS

FROM THE EDITORS OF *COSMOPOLITAN*

CHRONICLE BOOKS

SAN FRANCISCO

Text copyright © 2017 by Hearst
Communications, Inc.
Photographs/Illustrations copyright
© 2017 by Hearst Communications, Inc.
All rights reserved. No part of this book
may be reproduced in any form without
written permission from the publisher.

Library of Congress
Cataloging-in-Publication Data available.

ISBN 978-1-4521-6340-6

Manufactured in Hong Kong.

Cover design by Allison Weiner
Cover illustrations by Jenny Yuen

COSMOPOLITAN
Creative Director: Theresa Griggs
Editor: Marina Khidekel
Writer: Julie Vadnal
Designer: Kristen Male
Illustrations: Jenny Yuen
Project Manager: Emily C. Johnson
Copy Editor: Ester Brooke Friedman

HEARST BOOKS
VP, Publisher: Jacqueline Deval

Cosmopolitan and Cosmo are trademarks
of Hearst Communications, Inc.

10 9 8 7 6 5 4 3 2 1

Chronicle books and gifts are available
at special quantity discounts to
corporations, professional associations,
literacy programs, and other organizations.
For details and discount information,
please contact our premiums department
at corporatesales@chroniclebooks.com
or at 1-800-759-0190.

Chronicle Books LLC
680 Second Street
San Francisco, California 94107
www.chroniclebooks.com

CONTENTS

HELLO, SEXY!

First, there was the *Kama Sutra,* the ancient Indian sex manual. Then came the *Cosmo Kama Sutra,* which gave some of those classic moves our own sultry spin. Now, we're bringing you this epic, all-new collection of eyebrow-raising and enlightening moves—101 sweet, sexy, so-*Cosmo* positions guaranteed to take your lust to the next level.

A sex life worth savoring involves experimenting as a couple—with different moves, toys, and mind-sets—because it's all too common to fall into the rut of relying on just a few trusty positions. (Who hasn't been guilty of that?) This must-own manual is packed with poses and toy suggestions that will drive both of you wild in surprising ways—and keep your passion burning bright. And because we know how important your pleasure is, we'll help you discover the sexy ideas, words, and scenarios that will put you in the mood to play and help you achieve the incredible orgasms you deserve. (*Psst:* Sometimes, it's the subtle little differences in positions that bring huge new sensations!) So if you're ready to mix it up, we've got you covered. On these pages, you'll find amazing positions like the Big Bend (page 29), which maximizes your pleasure, the Stroke Show (page 62), which gives him a killer view of your bod that he'll bank in his memory forever, and the Work-It Wheelbarrow (page 171), which takes you both out of your physical comfort zones and boosts your bond—and your triceps!—in the process.

You in? We thought so!

Just like with good sex, there's no right or wrong way to do it (by which we mean diving into this book). Flip through with your partner—our 50 super-steamy Sex Challenges should keep your carnal calendar full for months. You could also bring it along to your next bachelorette bash and test your sexual intelligence against your friends'—our eye-opening Hot Topics give you the *Cosmo*-approved scoop on everything from advanced kissing maneuvers to extra-special oral techniques to a bit more risqué kinky sex. Or keep the book by your bedside to brush up on your skills for when you meet a hot new partner. To help guide you, each position falls within a category that indicates its carnal challenge level: Sweet and Sexy, Super Steamy, and for the truly adventurous, Burn the Sheets! No matter how you read it, we promise that after sinking your teeth into our ultimate collection, your sex life will never be the same.

—THE EDITORS OF *COSMO*

PART 1

SWEET AND SEXY

IS IT JUST US, OR IS IT GETTING TOASTY IN HERE? WHETHER YOU'RE EASING IN WITH SOMEONE NEW OR REVISITING THE CLASSICS WITH YOUR LONGTIME LOVE, THESE FOOLPROOF FAVES WILL RAISE YOUR TEMPERATURE IN NO TIME.

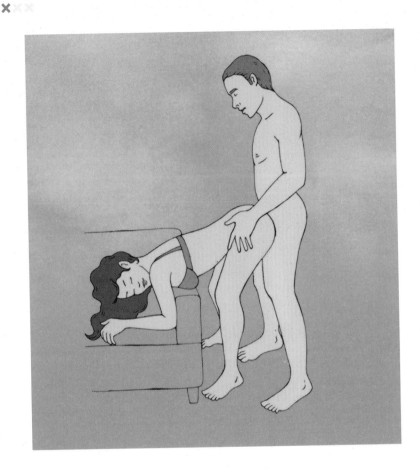

Sofa Squeeze

During your next Netflix and chill sesh, bend over the arm of the couch and lean your elbows onto the seat cushion so that your head slopes downward while he enters you from behind. The elevated angle means he'll hit you deeper than an episode of *The Wire*. Just don't forget to hit pause on the remote first.

SWITCH IT UP: **Place a throw pillow under your elbows to straighten your back and keep blood from rushing to your head. Now it'll only rush to your hoo-ha as the sex gods intended.**

Super-Close Cuddle

Add even more intimacy to missionary by wrapping your legs around his waist and crossing your ankles. Not only will the extra closeness give you tons of hot skin-on-skin contact, but also the upward angle of your hips gives him a direct route to your G-spot. It's like a hug, but way hornier.

MAKE IT HOTTER: **You're already face-to-face. Now make out like your tongues are long-lost BFFs.**

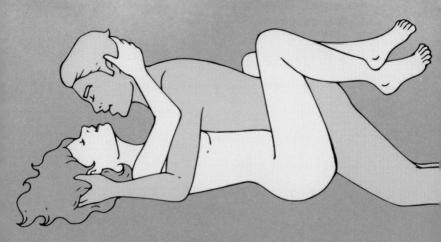

Begin your erotic activities by taking turns giving each other massages—starting at your shoulders and working your way down to . . . *not* your shoulders. Then let the ravaging begin.

Mattress Mash-Up

Move aside your pillows and lie flat on your stomach with your legs spread open about halfway as he stretches his body over yours, resting his elbows and legs on either side of you, then enters you from behind. Get ready for some crazy-deep penetration—the kind you'll have sweet, sweet dreams about.

NEXT-LEVEL IT: **As he thrusts, close your legs so your thighs touch. The extra tightness will make him feel king-size inside you.**

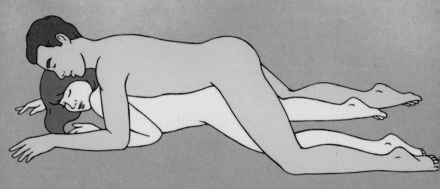

KISSING

Because some key lip-on-lip skills can take an ordinary hookup to new heights!

HOW TO GET HIM TO KISS THE WAY YOU WANT

Gently hold his face still, tell him to stop moving, and let him simply receive your kisses for a minute. That way, he'll know just how to kiss you back.

HOT PLACES TO KISS HIM . . . THAT AREN'T HIS LIPS

> Ears
> Eyelids
> Shoulders
> Chest
> Nipples
> Adonis belt
(that hot V-line his hip bones make—it's super sensitive for him!)

Three Kisses to Try Tonight

THE SURPRISE SMOOCH
Mid make-out, suck on his tongue firmly for a quick second. The swiftness will surprise him— you'll practically see the thought bubble above him saying, "Uh, did that just happen?"— and the excitement will make him want S-E-X, like N-O-W.

THE LIP SERVICE
Switch up the intensity and speed of your make-out sesh by playfully nibbling on his lower lip and tugging it toward you. The little bit of roughness lets him know you're in the mood for an intense romp.

THE ON-THE-MOVE XO
Starting at his neck, give him quick fluttery pecks, varying your kisses on your way down to his boxer briefs. He'll be totally turned on while he wonders where you're going to kiss him next.

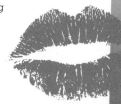

The Tsunami

Imagine your body is a surfboard and your man is lying on it, stomach-down. While he shimmies up your body a few inches, start having sex with him thrusting down and inward, then up and outward, giving your clit a tsunami wave of amazingness.

MAKE IT HOTTER: **Gaze into each other's eyes while you're doing the deed—you'll instantly feel more connected.**

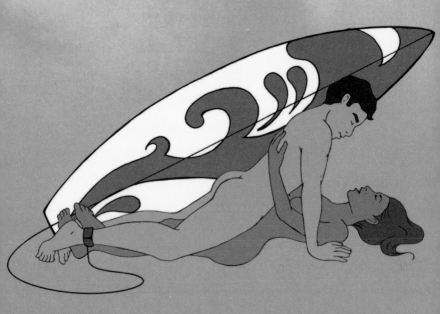

Simulate sex during foreplay by sucking his fingers or sliding his hand back and forth between your breasts. The suggestion of what's to come will have you both bursting at the seams.

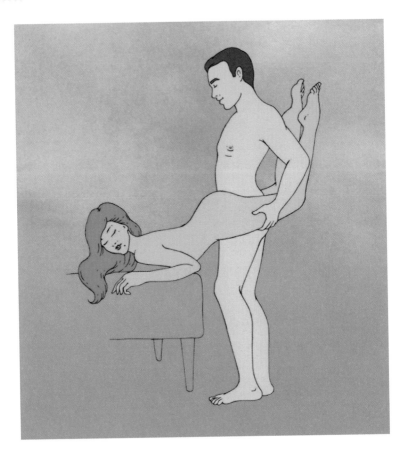

The T-Bone

For this sizzler, lie on the bed facing down with your legs hanging off the side. He'll stand behind you and hold your legs while he thrusts away, giving Michelin-star service to your G-spot. Bon appétit!

NEXT-LEVEL IT: **Complement your main dish by using one of your free hands to stroke your clitoris.**

No-Hands Nookie

While he's lying down, take charge and insist he keep his hands above his head. Tell him he's not allowed to move until you say so. Then lick and stroke up and down his body until you feel like getting on top. Once you're on him, caress your breasts, tummy, and clitoris, swatting away his hands . . . until you decide he can finally touch.

MAKE IT HOTTER: **Bind his hands up together with his tie or a scarf from your closet. Only let him free when he begs.**

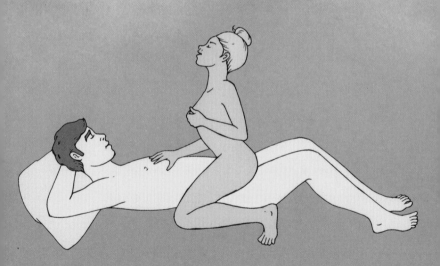

Send him this text and this text only: "I need you now." Don't be surprised when your doorbell rings approximately five seconds later.

Swirl'd Peace

Give doggie a new spin by placing his hand on your clitoris while he moves his hips in circles inside you. (You can guide him by moving your hips in a circular motion too.) The extra sensations mean you'll reach nirvana in record time.

NEXT-LEVEL IT: Instead of having him use his hands, hand him a bullet vibe for a high you'll barely be able to handle. Barely.

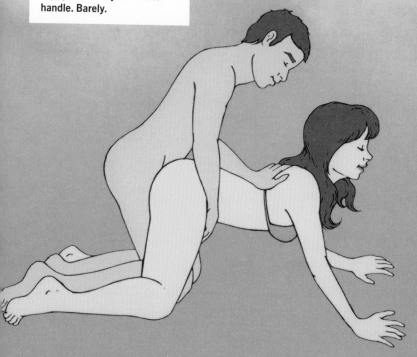

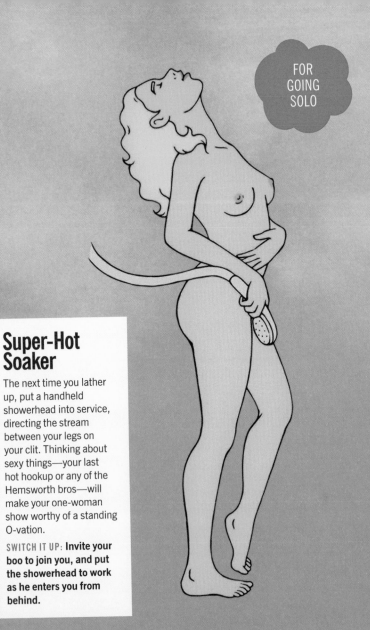

Super-Hot Soaker

The next time you lather up, put a handheld showerhead into service, directing the stream between your legs on your clit. Thinking about sexy things—your last hot hookup or any of the Hemsworth bros—will make your one-woman show worthy of a standing O-vation.

SWITCH IT UP: **Invite your boo to join you, and put the showerhead to work as he enters you from behind.**

The next time you're both whipping up dinner, stir things up by wearing lacy lingerie—and nothing else!—under your apron. It's a classic for a reason. (Also, every chef worth her salt knows that countertops are the perfect height for some oral sex on you.)

23

ANTICIPATION

Sure, intercourse gets all the glory, but the lead-up should be just as hot as the main event. Because epic sex starts with great sexpectations.

TEASE HIM IN THE A.M.

Roll over in the sheets and start a feverish make-out session. Just when he thinks he's getting morning sex, pull away and say, "We'll finish this tonight," and bounce out the door. By night-time, you'll both be ready to pick right back up where you left off.

SNAP SEXY SELFIES

Throughout the day, send him pics of your hot-ass self, starting from the ankles up, then from the collar-bone down. Just when he thinks he's gonna get a money shot, text him that he's now got a road map for his mouth to follow tonight.

SEND HIM AN INVITE TO PLAY

Send him the sexy evening itinerary as iCal invites. Shoot him an appointment for an 8 p.m. oral on him, then request that he return the favor at 8:15. Block off an hour for a "mind-blowing sex session." Then cap it off with a 9:30 snuggle sesh. He'll never accept a meeting invite faster.

The *Very* Good Morning

Start the day by lying on your stomach and letting him slide in from behind with his knees bent and arms supporting his weight at your sides. After sharing a bed all night, your bodies will be relaxed and ready for each other (especially his because of the glories of morning wood) and since you're facing away from him, no worries about the non-glories of morning breath.

MAKE IT HOTTER: **No pressure to exert too much energy in the a.m.—move a hand down to your clit for double the feels and half the effort.**

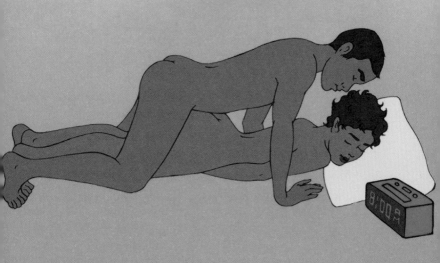

Breast Picture

Set your guy on a chair and climb aboard so your boobs are at mouth level. Sitting on top of him like this gives him perfect tongue access to those award-worthy beauties of yours. Run a nipple across his lips, then let him lick or suck as you bounce slowly up and down.

NEXT-LEVEL IT: Use your free hands to massage the back of his head . . . . He'll think he died and went to heaven.

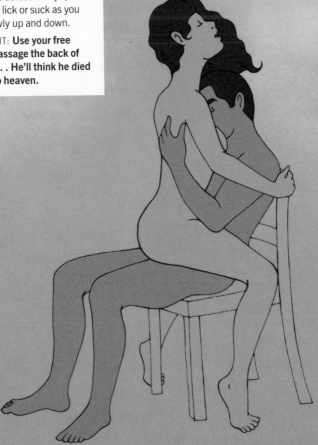

While he's going down on you, tell him to insert a finger and stroke your G-spot with a come-hither motion. The double stimulation will give you The. Best. O. Of. Your. Life.

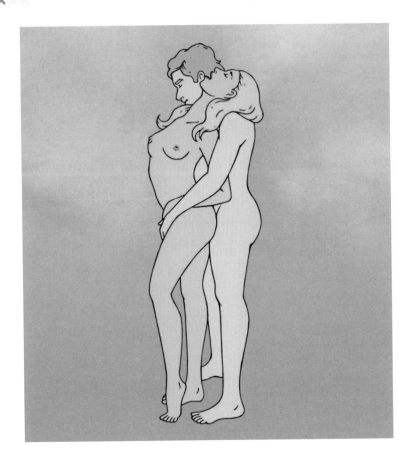

Party of Two

It's easy to get stuck on the idea that sex = P-in-the-V only. But sex is so much more than that. Try this intimate twist: With him standing behind you, he can alternate between stroking himself while you attend to yourself and touching you while he slides his Oscar Mayer Wiener between your hot buns.

MAKE IT HOTTER: **Take your two-person show to the shower, where he can rub himself against your soapy body.**

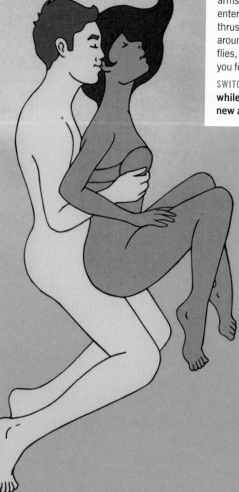

Big Bend

Get in a spooning position but curl up into more of a ball. Have him wrap his arms around you (how sweet!) and enter you from behind with long slow thrusts. The intimacy of his arms around you will make you feel butterflies, and the G-spot action will make you feel, well, something more intense!

SWITCH IT UP: **Uncurl out of your ball while he speeds up his thrusts. Those new angles are the stuff of greatness.**

Trace your hand along the inside seam of his jeans at the movies, or "accidentally" brush your booty against him in the elevator. Nothing is sexier to a guy than knowing you can't wait to rip off his clothes.

Invisible Man

Pop a dildo on a chair or the floor, kneel above it, and lower yourself onto it while holding it with one hand. Keep your stance wide for insane G-spot stim, or position your knees close for a tighter feel. Even if you don't O with just penetration (like practically everyone, although lube helps!), it can feel damn good to be in total control.

MAKE IT HOTTER: Once you've perfected your back and forth (or up and down, whatever!), add a pebble vibe to the mix to make your clit a part of the action too.

FOR
GOING
SOLO

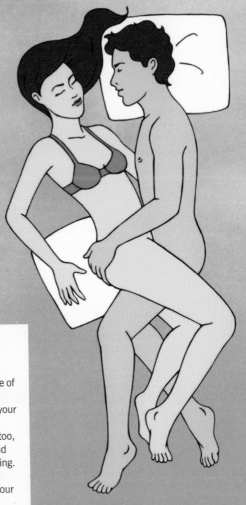

The Corkscrew

Turn missionary on its side by placing a pillow under one side of your butt and back so your shoulders are on the bed but your lady parts are pointing in his direction. He'll lie on his side too, as you intertwine your legs and let him take care of the thrusting. The twist in your body means you'll really feel him against your clit—hello, lazy girl's O!

SWITCH IT UP: **The same move, but this time you're lying on your side and he's doing the twisting. Wrap your legs around his torso for even more intimate sexin'.**

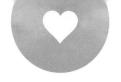

After a shower while the bathroom's still steamy, get him to take you from behind while you're leaning over the sink and pressing your hand against the fogged-up mirror, *Titanic*-style.

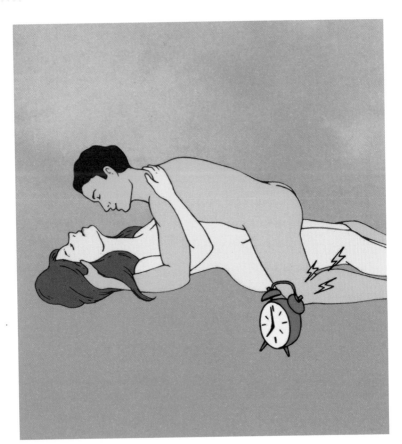

The Wake-Up Call

On a lazy Sunday when you #CantEven, press your legs together in missionary and, *whoa*, every move will be seriously enhanced. It's like a sexy version of a shot of espresso. And if your guy is on the smaller side, he will feel like he's filling you up and won't slip out. Good morning!

NEXT-LEVEL IT: **Roll your hips around slowly and you'll get this amazing slide-y friction that's so much more fun to wake up to than an alarm clock.**

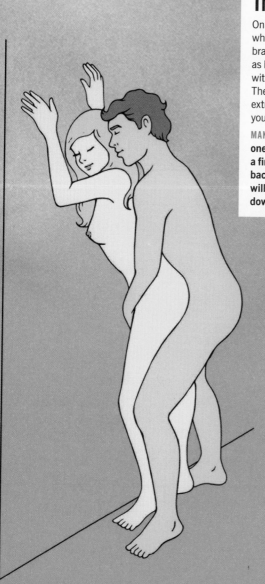

The Warm-Up

On a chilly winter night—or when the AC is on full blast—brace yourself against a wall as he enters you from behind with help from warming lube. The heated sensations and extra G-spot feels will make you both melt.

MAKE IT HOTTER: He can use one of his free hands to drag a finger up and down your back. The chills you'll get will go nicely with the heat down below.

Instead of simultaneously 69-ing, take turns. Get into position—but let one person go to town while the other groans and moans about how good it feels. Then switch!

LET'S (ACTUALLY) TALK ABOUT SEX

Carnal convos *can* be sexy . . . we promise!
Here's how to play it cool.

TRY THIS LINE

"I want to be your best ever, and I'm gonna need to study up. So tell me: What gets you going?"

TURN IT INTO A GAME

While lying in bed, take turns thinking of sexual scenarios (threesomes? sex in public?) and sharing whether it's a yes/no/maybe for each other. It's a game that's actually fun, and it's a low-key way to cover a lot of ground.

HIGHLIGHT THE GOOD STUFF

Every time you guys have sex, do a quick post-coital post-mortem by sharing your moves. ("When you cupped my ass!" "When we were moving in sync right toward the end!") Skip any critiquing because people tend to be sensitive after they've just been so intimate. Positive reinforcement means he's way more likely to repeat the action . . . and maybe go for round two?

Self-Reflection

Kneel in front of a full-length mirror and slide your hands over your breasts—squeezing, massaging, maybe a little pinching . . . basically figuring out what you like. Move your hands down your stomach to your inner thighs and your ladyflower. Watching yourself get turned on is *such* a turn-on.

NEXT-LEVEL IT: **Try it with a couple of pumps of flavored lube. Can't get yummier than that.**

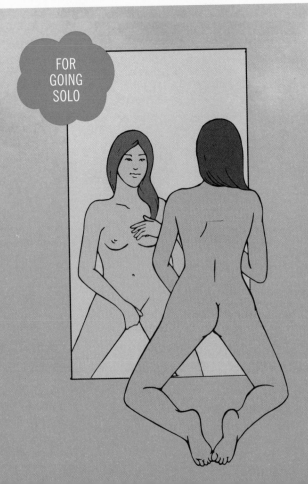

FOR
GOING
SOLO

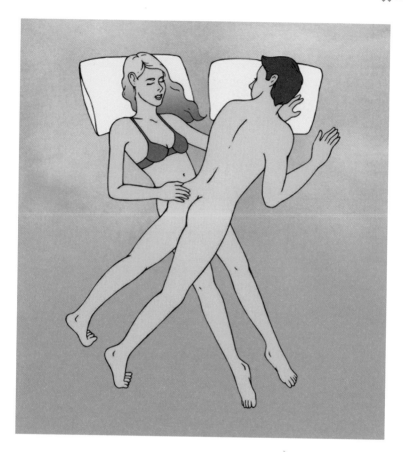

X Marks the Spot

In missionary, adjust yourselves so he's 45 degrees to one side and your bodies are making an X. At this sideways angle, the penetration will be shallow—good news for your clit . . . and even better news for guys with supersize sausages.

SWITCH IT UP: **Right before you're about to O, have him twist to the other side and get the good feels there too.**

The next time you're watching live TV (we know, rare), try "commercial sex." Start getting it on during the commercial, then untangle as soon as the show comes back. The teasing will be more suspenseful than a Shonda Rhimes plotline.

The S.S. Sexy

All aboard! Fill up the tub halfway and loll in his arms while he's entering you from behind. The water makes you weightless, so he can rock you for what seems like forever—although if you haven't found your sea legs yet, grab onto the edges of the tub for stability. (Extra important when you're about to O!)

MAKE IT HOTTER: **Because H$_2$O can make you dry (ironic, no?), rub down your sea captain with a silicone-based lube, which works in water.**

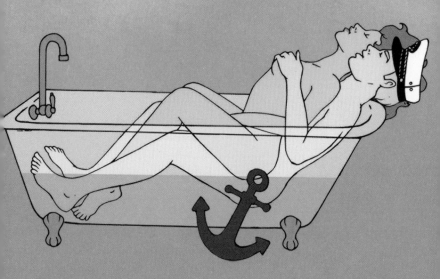

Ping Me

Kneel and lean down over a stack of pillows while he kneels and leans on you from behind, his legs outside of yours. As he thrusts, you're getting G-spot action, lazy intimacy, and free hands to grab your iPhone and check your e-mail. JK! JK?

NEXT-LEVEL IT: **Play with the number of pillows to adjust the angle of his penetration, adding new sensations.**

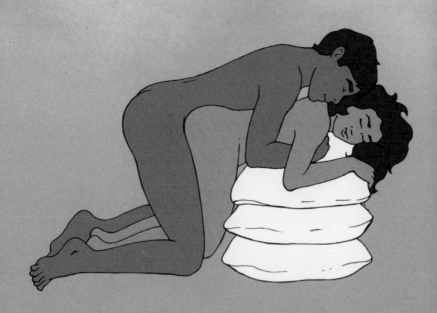

Slip off your panties—
but keep your skirt
on!—for girl-on-top
sex. So demure . . .
but, like, totally not.

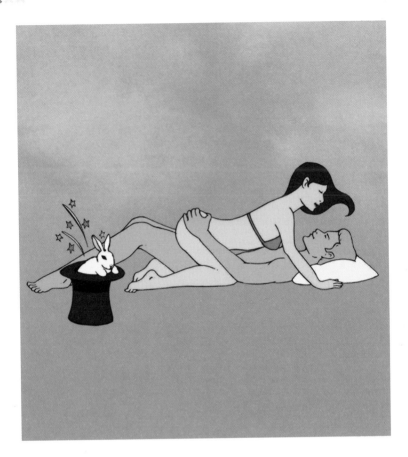

Magic Mash-Up

For your next trick, get on top with your upper body flush against his, and rock gently in whatever way feels most magical for you. You'll love the pelvic friction so much that—presto!—you'll O in no time. Plus, your breasts against him will make him feel like he'll never want you to disappear.

MAKE IT HOTTER: **Moving your hips in slow circles while you're on top will make a seriously sexy impact on his wand.**

The Pillow Fort

For an uplifting new take on missionary, place two pillows under your booty while he kneels and enters you. The altered point of entry will make you (and your G-spot) feel like you've invented a whole new kind of action, and he'll be free to thrust away at any pace.

SWITCH IT UP: **Add two more pillows—you know you own them—under your shoulders too, so you're flat, but your body is higher than usual. Then let him thrust straight on.**

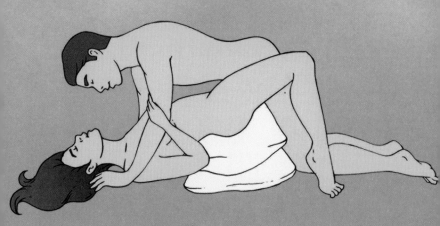

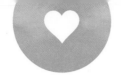

When you're going down on him, put the tip of your tongue against the roof of your mouth, so his shaft hits the underside of your tongue, making it feel like you're taking him all the way in.

Morning Glory

During those lazy early-morning hours, lie on top of him in your bed, both of you facing up, while he enters you from behind. He can gently rock you up and down as you use a bullet vibe on yourself. The combo of minimal effort and maximum clitoral action will definitely brighten up breakfast.

NEXT-LEVEL IT: **Place his hands on your breasts for a little daylight delight.**

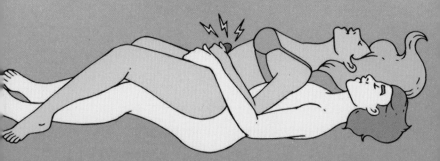

Pickle Tickle

Sit on his thighs with your legs out wide. Slide your hips back and forth, stimulating the sensitive first few inches of your vagina with the head of his penis. Take your time to enjoy all the glories of shallow penetration, which is also ideal for XL cucumbers.

MAKE IT HOTTER: **Lean back on your hands to deepen the penetration and give your G-spot some lovin'.**

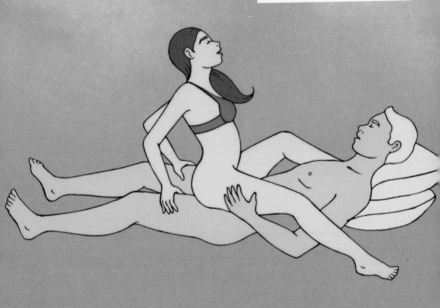

Get sex on the brain by reading a romance novel before a hot date night. The story will help you feel more sensual during the night as you recap the hottest scenes in your head.

SELF-LOVE

One is not the loneliest number.
Actually, solo action puts you
in touch with your turn-ons, which
makes you way better for sex
with someone else.

3 Ways to Get Yourself in the Mood

1.

Seduce yourself by gently stroking
your erogenous zones: your inner thighs,
behind your knees and ears, and the
nape of your neck. Instant heat.

2.

Burn a scented candle to warm
yourself up—according to the Smell and
Taste Treatment and Research Foundation
in Chicago, Illinois, lavender and
pumpkin pie aromas increase vaginal
blood flow by 11 percent.

3.

Pull up a hot scene from a
movie—even *The Notebook* works
here—on your laptop. Getting
mentally turned on will make you feel
instantly hotter.

How to Host a Party of One

DON'T LIMIT YOURSELF
Sure, all the women in movies masturbate
while lying on their backs, but if you
had your first O grinding on a couch
cushion, flip yourself over and get down
with a down pillow.

BE A TEASE
Bring yourself close to O in your
go-to style (clitoral stroking after a glass
of sauv blanc?), stop, and start again.
Big suspense = bigger orgasm.

CURE BUZZ BOREDOM
Using the same porn/vibe/position
every time? Try a masturbation
cleanse. Going back to basics can
make for a powerful O.

YAY FOR KEGELS!
The vaginal-clenching exercises
can lead to a stronger orgasm and serve
as training for the mythical hands-
free orgasm. Remind yourself to train
daily with a Kegel exercise.

KILL TWO Os WITH ONE TOY
Treat yourself to a dual-action vibe.
The smaller end fits inside you for G-spot
feels while the wider end buzzes up
against your clit—you control the sensations
with the handy remote.

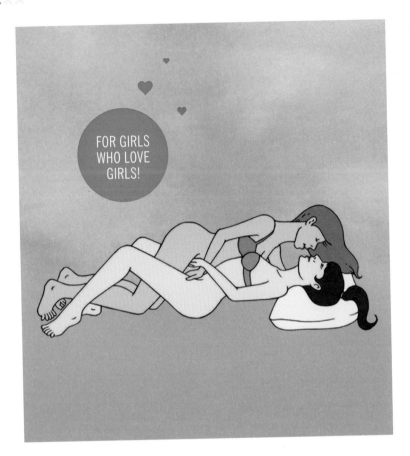

FOR GIRLS WHO LOVE GIRLS!

The Two-Way Touch

Lie on top of your lady and penetrate each other with your fingers simultaneously. Even though you're only using your hands, your bodies will be close for some super-connected breast-on-breast action and serious making out.

NEXT-LEVEL IT: **Follow her lead with her movements—when she gives you a come-hither finger, do the same. Following the leader never felt so rewarding.**

Erotic Embrace

Kneel, facing each other. Wrap one leg around his waist, and tilt your pelvis up, working your pelvic-floor muscles and increasing blood flow to your hoo-ha in the process. This super-intimate position (it's basically one super-hot hug) is best if you're near the finish line.

SWITCH IT UP: **When he bends his knees and sits on his feet, the adjusted angle will make him feel deeper than the diving end of a swimming pool.**

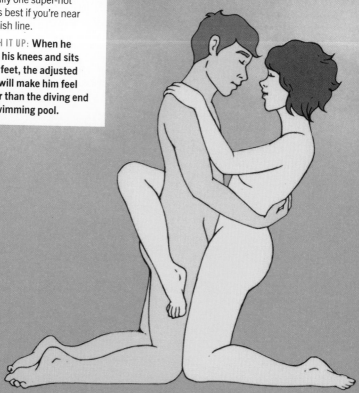

As you're getting into your foreplay groove, tell him to stop kissing you, and take over. This way you dictate the speed.

The Rocker

Straddle your guy with knees bent and toes touching the bed. Now rock back and forth like you have the tour bus all to yourselves. For a shallower ride, lean back and brace yourself. The head of his, um, microphone and first third of your vagina contain the most sensitive nerve endings, which means you'll both hit high notes.

NEXT-LEVEL IT: **Hold a bullet vibe against your clit and hand him the remote, which lets him control the buzzy patterns. It's like putting a playlist on shuffle and letting the good vibrations take over.**

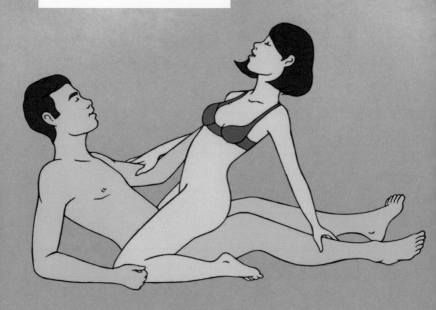

Over Easy

Lie on your back with both your legs up over your partner's shoulders while he penetrates you missionary style. With your bum elevated like that, you'll feel him super-deep, meaning your G-spot will get more love and praise than *Hamilton: An American Musical.*

SWITCH IT UP: **Instead of hooking both legs over his shoulders, take one down and leave it at his side. It's a serious stretch for you, but the sideways angle of your hips means even better feels.**

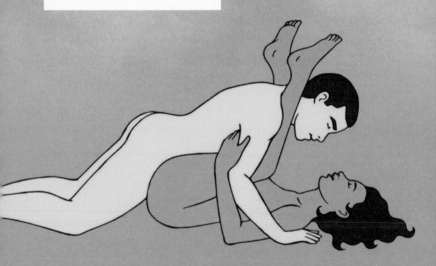

Ask him to trace his tongue over your thin-skinned spots: wrists, inner knees, behind your ears. It'll make you shiver.

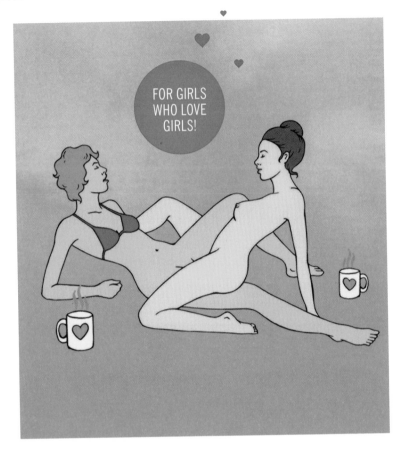

FOR GIRLS WHO LOVE GIRLS!

The Coffee Grind-Her

This girl-on-girl scissoring move is a classic for a reason. Straddle one of her legs so that your clits are aligned, then get to the grind. Moving your hips back and forth while you're on top gives you both some sweet on-and-off C-spot stimulation. It's so much more energizing than your morning latte run.

NEXT-LEVEL IT: **Adding a dime-size amount of lube into the mix will give whole new feels to synchronized hip swaying.**

The Lazy Girl's Beej

Lie on your sides facing each other, then slide down until his Johnsonville brat is all up in your grill. (Translation: His penis is near your face.) This position is the best way to give him pleasure without killing your knees or getting a major neck cramp.

MAKE IT HOTTER: While you're down there, use a hand to gently cup his balls up toward his body. It'll increase his sensations by a gazillion.

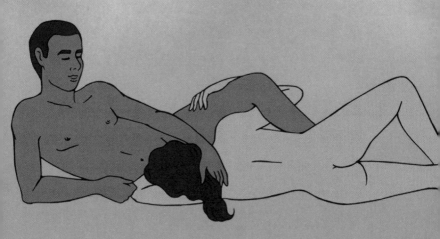

For every ten licks, take your mouth all the way up and off his package. Pause for a few agonizing beats to tease him with a smile before going back down.

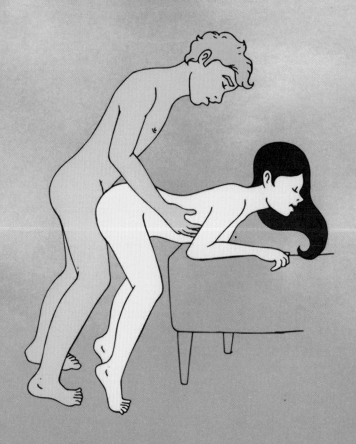

The Bed Spread

Lean over the edge of the mattress, presenting your ass fetchingly. He gets one hell of a view, and doggie-style lets him take you super deeply, using your hips for extra leverage. *Hello,* G-spot O!

MAKE IT HOTTER: **While he's thrusting behind you, give your girls some lovin' with your hands. Or just lie there and let him do the work. Because you deserve it.**

The Stroke Show

While giving him a VIP view of your booty in reverse-cowgirl, stay up on your knees for shallow strokes that'll stimulate the sensitive front third of your vagina (nearest the opening) and the nerve-packed tip of his penis.

SWITCH IT UP: **Once you're near the finish line, bring your booty closer to his tummy to go deep.**

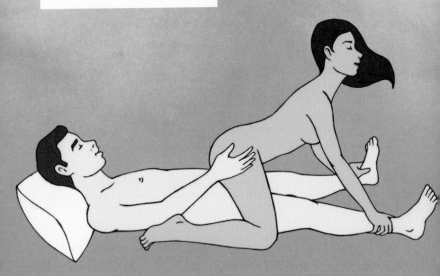

The next time
you're sexing, tell
your guy to skip
the in-and-out thrusts
and ask him to
stir with his penis.
The circular motion
will make you
(the good kind of)
dizzy.

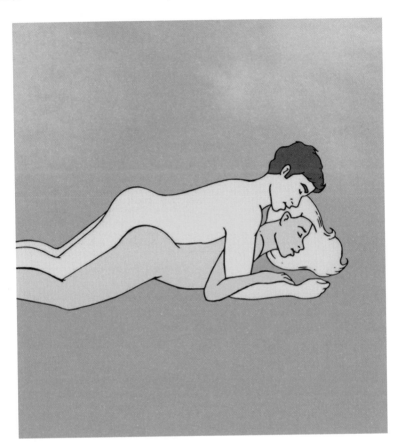

Floor Exercises

Hit the mat with your teammate, and lie facedown with your legs spread and him on top. (He'll support himself with his forearms.) As you rock slowly, his weight adds pressure on your G-spot. Take your time with this one. G-spot orgasms are a marathon, not a sprint.

NEXT-LEVEL IT: **Go for the gold and bring your legs together as he thrusts. The tightened positioning is one you'll both double-flip for.**

Mount O-lympus

Kneel and slope downward as much as possible keeping your legs together while your Eros (the Greek god of love) grabs your waist. Pressing your thighs together works the pelvic muscles, making you feel like the goddess of amazing orgasms.

MAKE IT HOTTER: **This is the perfect position to achieve a double-stimulation O with a pebble vibe—it's the stuff legends are made of.**

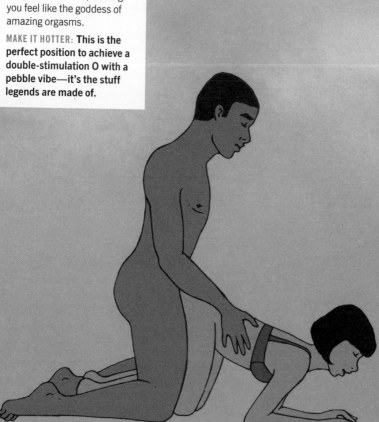

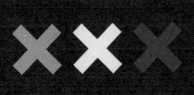

PART 2

SUPER
STEAMY

YOU'VE MASTERED THE BASICS. NOW IT'S TIME TO CRANK
UP THE HEAT ON YOUR LOVEMAKING GAME. JUST
REMEMBER TO STAY HYDRATED—SOME OF THESE MOVES
COULD DOUBLE AS A VERY SEXY WORKOUT.

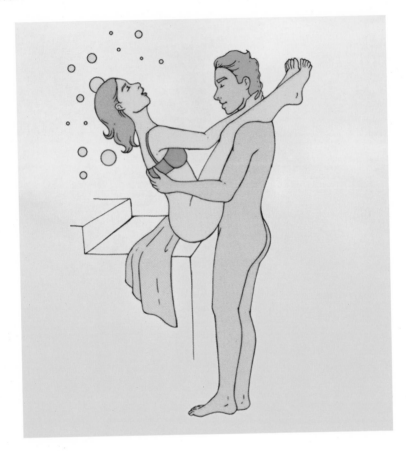

The Spin Cycle

Sneak off to your laundry room and sit on the dryer while your man stands and faces you. Turn on the dryer so it vibrates while he's entering you, and put your legs over his shoulders so you'll feel every bit of his, um, load.

NEXT-LEVEL IT: Sure, your clothes will be getting dry, but a couple drops of lube will keep you anything but.

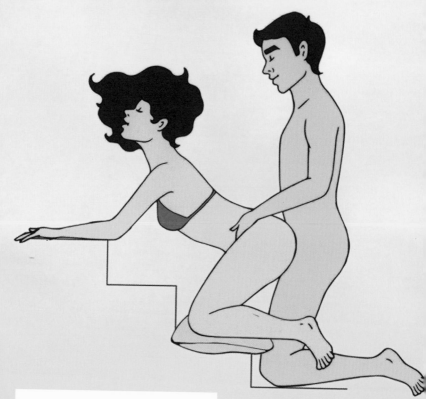

Stairway Sizzler

Kneel in front of your partner at the landing of a staircase so that you're a step or two above him. (Don't go too high up, because, well, safety, and place your just-discarded dress or his jeans under your knees so you have a cushion.) Place your hands on a higher step for support while he holds your hips and gives your G-spot some step-by-step stimulation.

SWITCH IT UP: **Lean into the steps to let him go even deeper. [Insert "Stairway to Heaven" reference here.]**

While your guy's still sleeping, get on top of him stark naked and pepper his face with light kisses to wake him up. Then press your body hard against him and begin inching his boxers down his hips. He'll be up and at 'em in no time.

The Giddyupper

While he's lying on his back with one leg bent, straddle his body backward, reverse-cowgirl style, and lower yourself onto his loyal steed. Press against his leg for clitoral stim as you're riding him for a gallop you'll both enjoy.

NEXT-LEVEL IT: **You'll have primo access to his crown jewels, so take the opportunity to play with them gently. Guys love a little attention to their sexy saddle bags during the deed.**

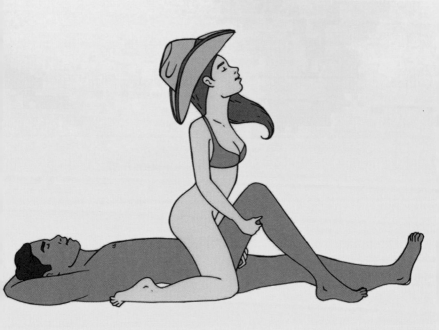

Spanks a Lot

As he sits up with his legs extended, straddle him in reverse but with your legs extended behind him and your torso down between his thighs and shins. He'll love the unforgettable rear view and how easy it is for him to gently smack your butt.

MAKE IT HOTTER: Amp things up by telling him to tug on your tresses a little too. All that power will give him a rush.

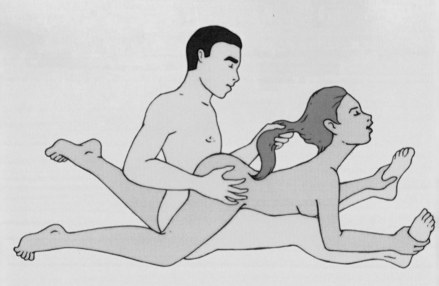

Keep your panties on during foreplay. He can massage you through the fabric— with his hands or his mouth—and send his anticipation through the roof.

DIRTY TALK

Yes, it's possible to whisper
naughty things without sounding
like you're auditioning for a
walk-on role in a *Fifty Shades* sequel.
Here's how to talk the talk.

How to Talk Dirty Without Sounding Ridiculous

START SIMPLE

You don't have to start spouting filthy
things right away. "Mmms" and "Oh yeahs" are
easy entry points. Even a "That feels *sooo*
good" can seriously steam things up.

GAUGE HIS DIRTY-TALK THRESHOLD

If you're not sure how nasty to get, whisper, "What
would you like me to do to you? Details, please."
See what words he uses and how racy he's
willing to get and follow his lead.

ASK FOR WHAT FEELS GOOD

Any dude will tell you that there's nothing hotter
than a woman who knows what she wants in bed. Tell
him what hot things you want him to do to you.
And if he's already doing them, let him know how
much you're enjoying it all.

DON'T WORRY ABOUT SOUNDING SILLY

Because really, who else is going to hear you but him?

Take these foolproof phrases for a test run.

HOW ARE YOU SO GOOD AT THIS?

YOU'RE SO HARD.

I WANT TO DO BAD THINGS TO YOU.

I'M SO WET.

I CAN'T WAIT TO FEEL YOU INSIDE ME.

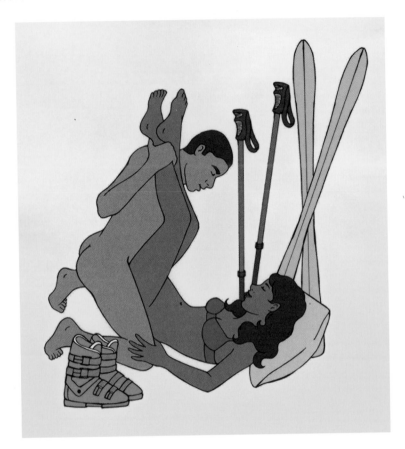

The Hot Ski Instructor

Keep your legs together (savvy skier style, natch) and lift them straight into the air. Lean them against one of his shoulders as he props up and leans forward, rubbing against your G-spot. Skiing is a downhill sport, but you're about to go up, up, and away.

NEXT-LEVEL IT: **Keep your socks on. Sounds crazy, but research shows that women are more likely to orgasm when wearing 'em. Cozy!**

The Sultry Short Stack

Slip yourself on top of your guy, aligning your bodies so that you're both facing the ceiling. (It's the perfect positioning for him to whisper dirty thoughts into your ear, just FYI.) While he thrusts slowly in and out of you, lift your hips up and down to control the penetration. You'll both melt faster than butter on French toast. Post-sex brunch, anyone?

MAKE IT HOTTER: **While he caresses your breasts with his free hands, use one of yours to make small, then wide, circles around your clit.**

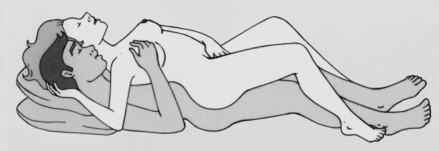

Usually get oral with your legs spread? Intensify your orgasm by stretching your legs straight out, stimulating the pelvic muscles that help you climax.

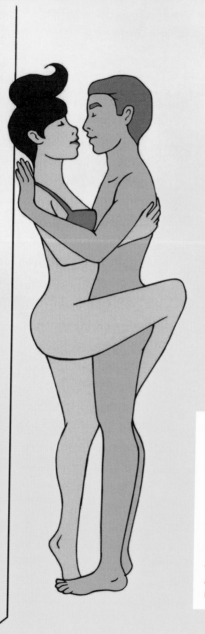

The Flamingo

Leaning against a wall and facing him, lift one leg and wrap it around his body while he enters you. The upward angle of your hips means he'll tickle your G-spot pink (like a flamingo, get it?).

SWITCH IT UP: **Stand on your tippy toes, which makes the angle of his thrusting even more O-mazing for you both.**

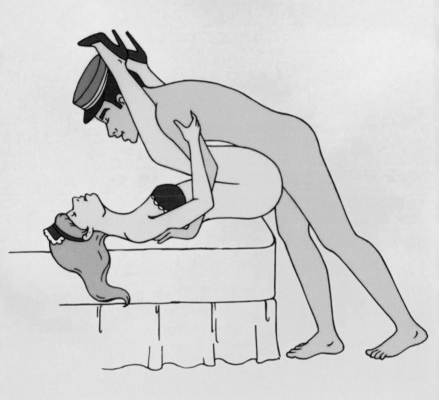

Do Not Disturb

The next time you're shacked up at a hotel, toss the hotel throw blanket to the side (gross) and put your booty at the edge of the bed. As he stands to enter you, put your legs over his shoulders and have him lean down between your legs. The deep feels will be so good that you won't even notice housekeeping knocking.

MAKE IT HOTTER: **Role-play. (Hotels are great for this!) He's the room-service delivery guy and you're the sexy maid? Adulterous lovers meeting for the first time? The whole thing is weirdly freeing because it's not you, it's your character.**

Push your breast friends up against your guy, then slide down his body with your nipples grazing his torso. The light touches will make him super hard.

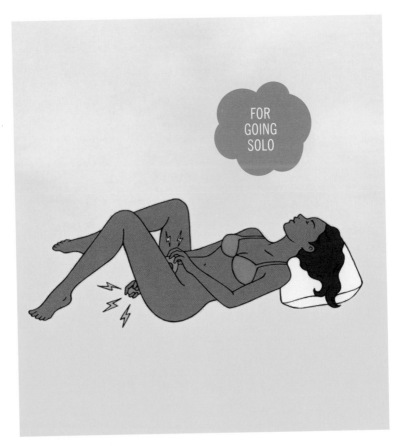

FOR
GOING
SOLO

The Electric Threesome

When it comes to solo sex, harness the power of three: you and two little friends. Start with an oral-sex simulator to work insanely perfect magic on your clit while you slide in a G-spot vibe. Double orgasm, anyone?

NEXT-LEVEL IT: **Try a vibe with suction powers for crazy-good clit feels. It's like a little BJ for your lady parts.**

Moaning Mermaid

Switch positions in missionary so you're on top, with your legs pressed together between his and your arms holding you up like Ariel on that rock. Since he's on the bottom, he can thrust extra deep inside you, and you'll get the clit-stimulating benefits of girl-on-top. Plus, the power reversal makes this feel a bit subversive . . . aka super hot.

MAKE IT HOTTER: **Stay extra still while he adjusts his thrusting by butterflying his legs wide and then bringing them closer together.**

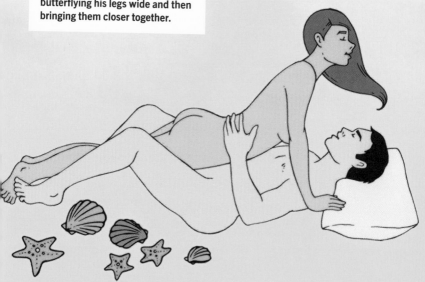

Keep your hand in constant motion on his shaft while you work him with your mouth, giving him the feeling of nonstop penetration.

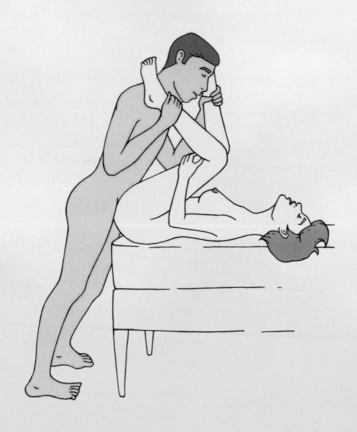

The Hello Cello

Bring your legs up to your chest and have him grab your ankles as he enters you. He can bend your legs, push them together on your chest, spread them apart, put them straight up—the challenge is figuring out exactly the right ways to play you, the instrument. The finale? An amazing O!

MAKE IT HOTTER: **Instruct him to go extra *slooow* with his movements. That way you'll be able to appreciate every angle of *his* instrument—and the anticipation will make you insanely hot.**

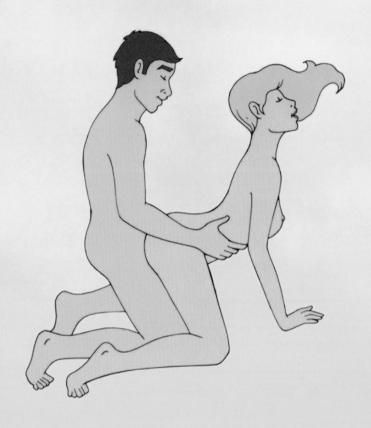

The Good Doggie

While he kneels behind you, get on all fours so he can hold your hips and thrust from behind. The genius to this classic positioning is all in the customization. Doggie-style is great for the less-endowed dudes because he can penetrate you more deeply so you get the most out of whatever he's packing—and you can further alter the feels for both of you by arching your back.

SWITCH IT UP: **Try resting your head all the way down on the bed until he's hitting you in exactly The. Right. Spot.**

Tap into a hot memory from your past that really lit your fire. Was it stress-free vacay sex? A hot session where you were so turned on, you didn't get to take your dress off? Try to recapture that same feeling tonight!

ORAL ON HIM

Forget good. Take our lead and he'll consider you epic.

THE STARTER BLOW JOB

Here's the basic rule to giving a great blow job: Use your mouth (obviously) and your hands. Your mouth is going to provide the sensation and lubrication (and for him, the all-important visual!), but your hands are going to do a lot of the work.

SO TRY THIS . . .

Take the head into your mouth and squeeze, lick, and swirl like you would a soft-serve cone. Meanwhile, use your hands to grip, squeeze, and stroke the length of his penis. Don't just keep doing the same motion—variety of sensation is key.

MIND THE STEPCHILDREN!

Cup and stroke his balls now and then—try pushing them up and (very gently) tugging them down.

THE CHERRY ON TOP?

Eye contact. Give a wink or some smize action and he'll be putty in your . . . mouth.

Advanced BJ Moves

ICE, ICE BABY

Playing with temperature
really feels amazing for him. If
your teeth are too sensitive
for the ol' ice-cube-in-the-cheek
trick, try alternating with
drinking something cold or warm.
Even easier, lightly blow
air over him after having had
him in your mouth.

THE CORKSCREW

Twist your hand as you
move up and down his shaft like
you're tracing the grooves
of a corkscrew and slide it over
his tip when you get to it. (Plenty
of lube is key for this move!)

THE TIP-OFF

The hole on his tip is called
the meatus, which is the
worst name ever given to
anything. But it's super sensitive
during arousal. With your
tongue, apply medium pressure,
on and off. He'll be shocked
at how good it feels.

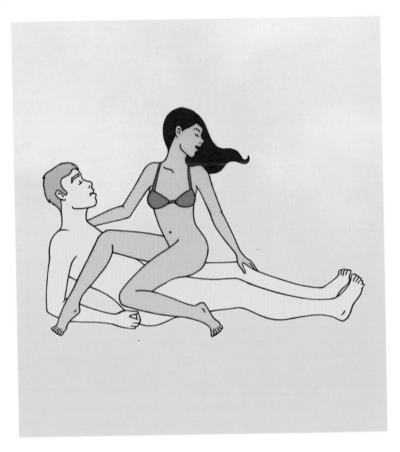

The Sexy Screw

Start on top, then when you're both about to lose your minds, swing your right leg over his torso—then your left over his legs—and swivel around to reverse-cowgirl, all while keeping him inside you. The switch-up is a fun surprise, and his new view will make him lose his mind all over again.

NEXT-LEVEL IT: **Once you're getting your grind on in reverse-cowgirl, switch back to girl-on-top. Full-circle sex!**

He's Hooked

While you're lying on your back, he kneels and sits to enter you, hoisting your hips onto his bent knees. Wrap your legs around his torso and hook your feet while he thrusts, giving you super-deep penetration that'll get you both— hook, line, and sinker.

MAKE IT HOTTER: **Use your free hands to pull his face closer to yours for some eye contact . . . then lip contact.**

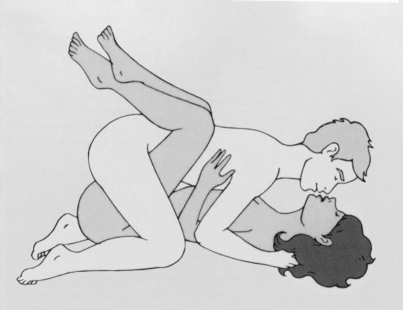

In an LDR? Send him a care package for his, um, package. Fill a box with some sexy new lingerie, a few condoms, some lube, and a sex toy. Send it to his front door with this note: "We'll need this on my next visit."

Steamy Slow Jam

It's like the Usher—or Marvin Gaye, or Monica, whatever you like—of sex positions. Lie on your side with him behind you, in spoon position. He lifts your leg and enters you from behind. The low-key action and intimate (aka *deeeep*) positioning let you both take your time to get there. Slow and steady wins the O-face!

SWITCH IT UP: **While your leg is in the air, he'll have an all-access pass to your clit. Let him rub with his fingers, or hand him a pebble vibe if you want to speed your jam up a little.**

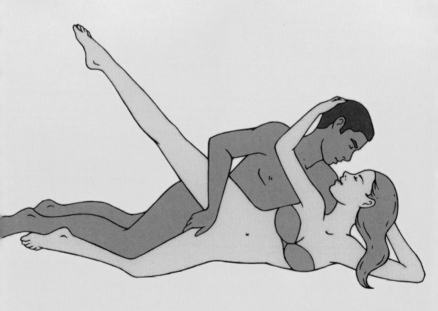

Headboard Hustle

Christen your new bed—or his for the first time—by lying on your back, while he kneels in front of you, pulling your legs straight up onto the top of his thighs. Brace yourself against your headboard (or wall) as he works his magic. You'll have to do your best not to wake the neighbors. (But, like, no promises.)

NEXT-LEVEL IT: Even though your hands will be above your head, his will be free to give your girls some love.

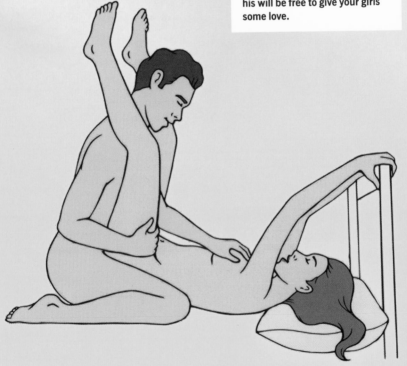

Lead with a compliment ("I love it when you . . .") before suggesting a new move. He'll never catch on that you're actually guiding him by saying, "And you know what else would turn me on? If you used two fingers right here." Shh! We'll never tell!

ORAL ON YOU

A hottie whose only goal is to make you moan with pleasure? We didn't think it was possible to make this move hotter, but here goes!

GETTING YOURSELF GOING

Most straight men enjoy going down on women, so you don't need to do much prep work. If you're one of the 37 percent of women who feels self-conscious about the way she smells or tastes, you can take a shower or use a wet-wipe beforehand. Close your eyes if it helps you turn off your brain. This is about *you*—so try to relax and enjoy it.

HELP HIM OUT

Talk to your partner. You can tell him what you like by affirming, "*Mmm,* like that," or offering something more specific like, "I love it when you circle my clit with the top of your tongue while touching me with your fingers."

DON'T BE AFRAID TO BE VOCAL

When he's going downtown, your pleasure is his goal. Show him with your hand where you want to be touched and the kinds of motions you like.

SHOW YOUR APPRECIATION

Whether it's through moans, body language, or a "Yes, keep going," men love a little direction. And the more positive feedback he gets, the more he'll want to do it again.

Give This to Your Guy!

Hand this oral-on-her primer to your partner. Then pat yourself on the back.

BE A TEASE

Give her quick kisses starting at her neck, circling her nipples, and trailing her stomach to her inner thighs. The anticipation will drive her Kanye-level crazy.

START SLOWLY

Begin with wide, slow licks up and down, followed by circles around her clit, so you hit all her hot spots. The buildup here is crucial for a shut-up-that's-so-good kind of O.

SHOW YOU'RE INTO IT

Tell her how gorgeous her [insert preferred lady-parts name] is. Or go, "God, you're beautiful." Flattery toward hoo-has goes a long way.

BE HANDSY

While you're down there, slide two fingers inside, faceup, then open and close them like you're making a peace sign. You'll hit her G-spot, that nerve-packed area just two inches inside the upper wall, and the double stimulation feels super groovy, baby.

GO VERTICAL

While you lie faceup, guide her to kneel above your head, facing you. While upright, she'll control your tongue's angle and pressure. And bonus: It's a starting point for some sweet, sweet 69.

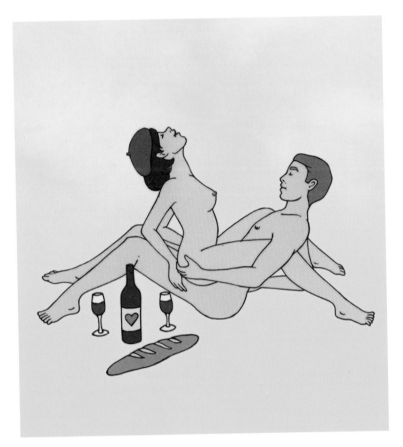

The French Kiss

Ready to say, "Oui! Oui!"? While he sits on the bed and leans backward, hook your legs over his hips, and lean back on your elbows. You won't have to do much work—French women don't really exercise, after all—but you'll still feel his baguette all up against your G-spot as you lazily grind. Berets not necessary, but what the hell?

MAKE IT HOTTER: Squeeze your pelvic-floor muscles (aka do some Kegels) just as he's about to . . . what's the French word for "totally lose it"?

Up and Down Doggie

Work your angles better than a Kardashian by propping your elbows on a pillow and lifting your butt high, tilting your pelvis to the heavens. Now he'll point his thrusts downward while you touch your clitoris. Geometry definitely wasn't this hot in high school.

SWITCH IT UP: **Straighten your arms and flatten your back to clench your stomach and pelvic muscles. Doing so right before you climax can make the sensation even more intense than usual.**

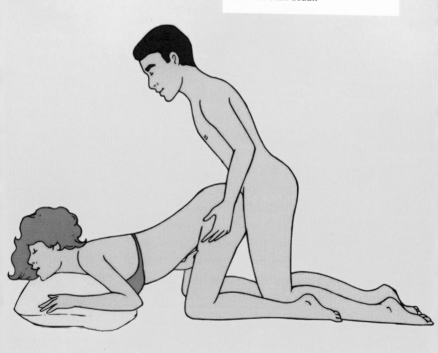

Sit behind him and use a finger to track zigzags across his shoulder blades and down his spine. The nerves along his lower back are directly connected to his package, so this will shoot currents of electricity between his legs.

Tug of Ween

Make like two horny summer campers and in reverse-cowgirl, give him your wrists and let him pull you toward him while you lean your body forward. Then let him win a little and arch your back so your labia majora rub a bit against his balls. Yes, it's a power play. But at sex camp, there can be two winners!

MAKE IT HOTTER: **Use a bandana to tie your hands behind your back. Giving yourself up and letting him take control can make you both _very_ happy bunkmates.**

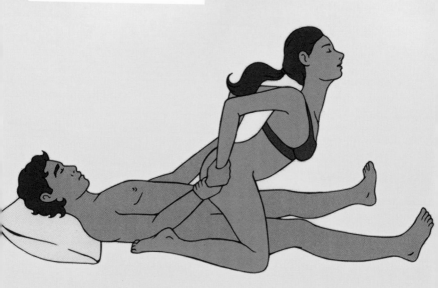

Rocket Raiser

For a missionary upgrade (emphasis on *up*), lie on your back and lift your legs to one side as he kneels and enters you. The squeeze and raise of your legs makes you super-tight, and the angle of your hips means he'll hit spots inside you that rarely get TLC. We have lift-off!

NEXT-LEVEL IT: **Let him play Mission Control by moving your hips left to right instead of in and out. The added G-spot stimulation will be out of this world.**

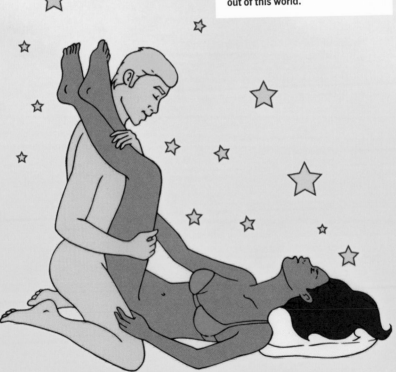

Trace the seam that runs down his testicles with your tongue. It's a nerve-packed pleasure area that's often overlooked, so he'll be Pharrell-style happy that you're down there.

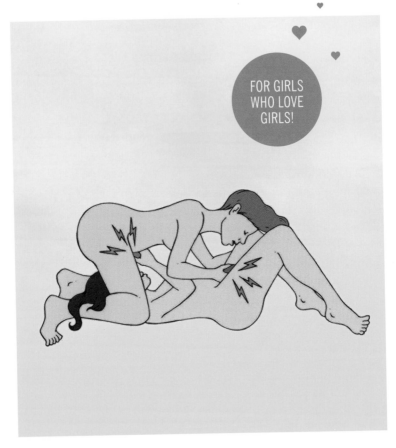

FOR GIRLS WHO LOVE GIRLS!

Electric 69

It's electric! Get in position for 69, but instead of using your tongues, use pebble vibes on each other. Play with the vibration patterns or get creative by making circles around her clit and varying the pressure—um, way more fun than being pulled into the Electric Slide at your cousin's wedding.

SWITCH IT UP: **Swap your external vibes with Rabbit-style ones that also have clit stimulators to double (er, quadruple!) the pleasure.**

The Tender Twist

Lie on your side, propping your upper body up with your arm. While he enters you from behind, rest your back thigh on his knee, keeping you nice and close. (It's also ample opportunity to get your kissing game on.) Enjoy the combo of rear entry and romance. *Awww . . .*

MAKE IT HOTTER: **Maintaining eye contact the entire time will make for an überclose, überhot experience you'll both be hard-pressed to forget.**

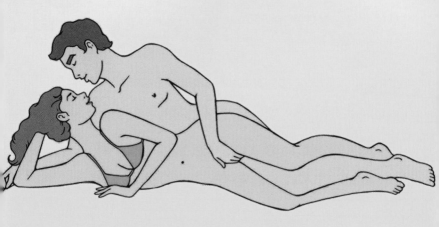

As he's pleasuring you down there, have him slip his hands under your butt and gently knead. Being stimulated from both sides enhances the sensation.

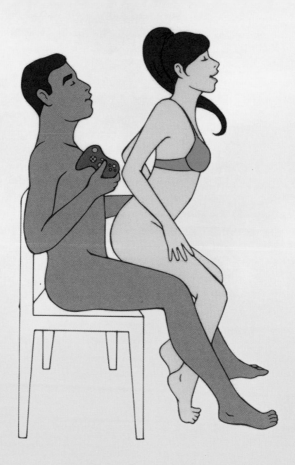

The XXX-Box Tourney

The next time he's in an Xbox trance, try a game where you'll both win. With your back to him, lower yourself down, pressing your legs together between his. Brace against his thighs and stick your booty back. From the depth to the angle, you'll take full control of his joystick.

NEXT-LEVEL IT: **Since you won't be facing each other, add some crazy-hot intimacy by inviting him to trace his fingers along your back, then move his hands around to the front, giving your nipples some fingertip action too. Score!**

You-and-Eye-Gasm

Straddle him and lean back until you're bracing your hands, connected only by your fun bits. Slowly move backward and forward. The combo of nerve-teasing shallow penetration—great for less-endowed fellas—and deep eye contact is sizzling.

MAKE IT HOTTER: **Invite a third party—a tiny bullet vibe—to your hot hang, and hand it to your guy to massage against your clit.**

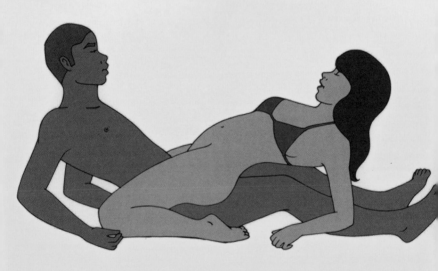

When you're close to orgasm, tighten and then relax your Kegels. This move alone can trigger a supercharged climax.

SEX TOYS

Whether you are looking to make
sex with bae even hotter or want to have
more fun flying solo, adding a
toy to the mix is always a good idea.

What's My Next Toy?

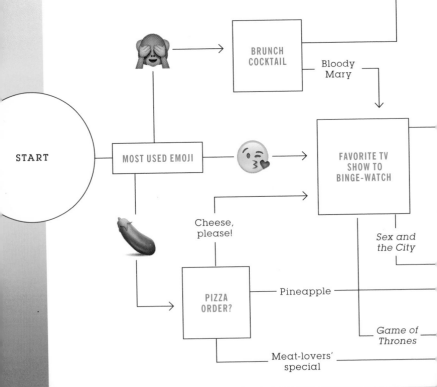

START

MOST USED EMOJI

BRUNCH COCKTAIL

Bloody Mary

FAVORITE TV SHOW TO BINGE-WATCH

Cheese, please!

Sex and the City

PIZZA ORDER?

Pineapple

Game of Thrones

Meat-lovers' special

Bellini ———————→

Drinks ———————→

BEGINNER
Pebble Vibe
The non-phallic shape of pebble vibes make them the least threatening things ever (a plus for dudes who may not have a lot of toy experience). But the strong vibrations and variety of settings render these babies serious threats . . . to your self-control.

IDEAL FIRST DATE

Rock climbing ———————→

iends

Surprise me!

INTERMEDIATE ←
Rabbit-Style Vibe
The long end of a classic Rabbit-style vibe buzzes against your G-spot while the "ears" massage your clit. If any toy can deliver a double orgasm, this is it!

SIGNATURE BEAUTY LOOK

Red lips ———————→

Smoky eye

ADVANCED
A Vibrating "Glove"
Go for a wearable vibe that's kind of like *Fifty Shades* meets *Iron Man*—a glove with finger pads that either vibrate or add little jolts of electrostimulation to wherever you (or your guy) touch.

CHIPS AND . . .?

Salsa . . . *picante!* ———————→

Guac ———————

Calling All
Sex Toy Shoppers!
Most retailers don't do returns
or exchanges . . . for obvious
reasons. Shop smart, or risk buying
a vibe that collects cobwebs.

ASK Q'S
"Where does this go?" and "What does
this button do?" are totally normal questions. Don't be
alarmed if a salesperson asks you some Qs
too. (They're not judging—promise!) Or if you're
shopping online, many sites let you live-
chat with a personal shopper.

TRY BEFORE YOU BUY
Okay, not literally because that would be gross,
but you should play with the buttons, see how the
vibrations feel in your hands, and test out all
the settings while you're still in the store. That's
what sample toys are for, so don't be shy.

LOOK BEYOND THE TRENDS
Everyone's bodies and sexual preferences are
varied, so what works for you might not work for a
friend. And just because you saw that one toy
on that one show once doesn't mean it has to be the
one you take home.

BRING FRIENDS!
Brunch and buzzfest, anyone? Shopping with
friends can make the whole experience less awkward
and more fun. Or if your boo is into it, make it a
fun daytime date that'll make both of you look forward
to that night. Getting an S.O.'s input can be
really helpful . . . and surprisingly sexy.

THE ONE EASY
SEX TOY TIP TO LIVE BY

Bring a bullet vibrator to
bed. The Rabbit gets all
the glory, but using a
bullet (or pebble) vibe
on your clit during
doggie is a game
changer.

HOW TO MIX SEX TOYS AND BOYS

It's understandable that dudes
who are new to toys might not
be obsessed with the idea.
Start with something that's not
peen-shaped, and guide
his hands exactly where it feels
good. He'll find your take-
charge attitude super sexy.

SHOPPING ONLINE?

Most stores and brands
offer discreet shipping
in plain brown boxes
with generic return
addresses to avoid any
awkward UPS sign-offs
or roommate run-ins.
Phew!

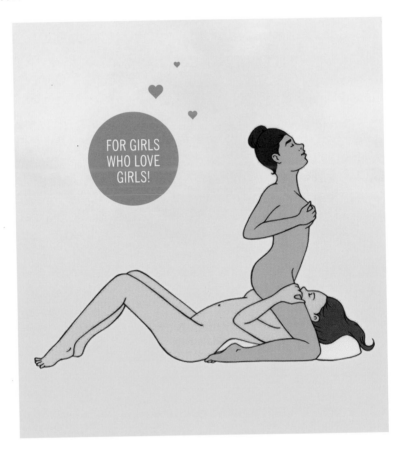

FOR GIRLS WHO LOVE GIRLS!

The Chart Topper

You know the Beyoncé song that starts, "Let me sit this *aaass* on you"? That's what you're going for here. Kneel over her shoulders and let your booty brush against her nipples while she gets intimate with your clitoris, making you hit Bey-level high notes.

NEXT-LEVEL IT: **Guide her toward what feels most amazing by shifting your hips forward and backward. Less work for her and more high notes for you.**

Sexy Stretch

Kneel with your feet under your booty and reach forward with your hands in front of you, like in child's pose (*ahhh*). Arch your hips as high as you can as he enters you from behind. This position may seem typical, but the direct action with your G-spot (and chance of an internal orgasm) is anything but.

SWITCH IT UP: **Give him a break from thrusting and rock your booty forward and backward while he stays still. Get it, girl.**

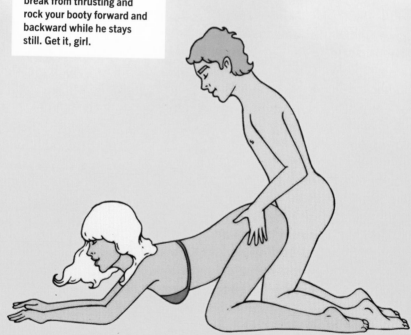

Perfect your striptease. Stage an entrance from another room, take a sensual walk around him, and slowly shed a slip to reveal a corset . . . or a thong . . . or if you're daring, nipple tassels! By the time you finally straddle him, you'll both be raring to go.

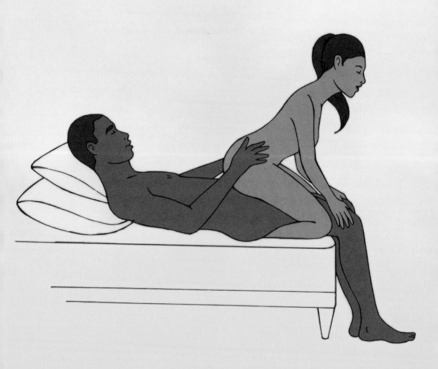

Edge of Glory

Take your sexing to the end of the bed for a slightly dangerous (okay, not really) turn. As he's lying on the edge of the bed, knees bent and feet on the floor, straddle him, facing away. Tuck your calves under his body for leverage as you ride him as quickly (or tantalizingly slowly) as you want.

NEXT-LEVEL IT: **Reach under and massage his perineum, which is such an intense pleasure center for him. You'll blow his mind! Give your clit some love with your other hand to bring you both over the edge.**

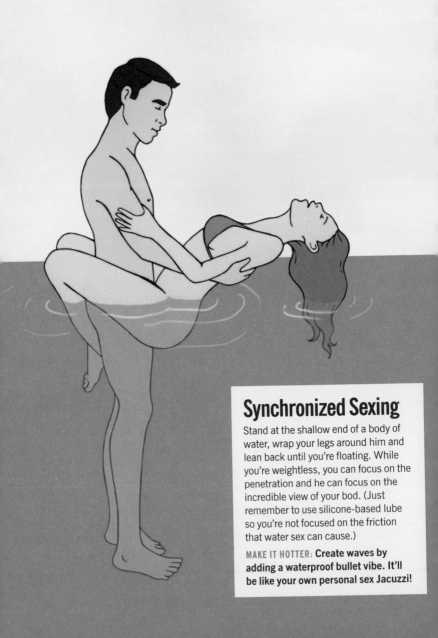

Synchronized Sexing

Stand at the shallow end of a body of water, wrap your legs around him and lean back until you're floating. While you're weightless, you can focus on the penetration and he can focus on the incredible view of your bod. (Just remember to use silicone-based lube so you're not focused on the friction that water sex can cause.)

MAKE IT HOTTER: Create waves by adding a waterproof bullet vibe. It'll be like your own personal sex Jacuzzi!

Show your guy
that you're aching
for him during sex.
It could be anything
from heavy breathing
to a soft moan,
even an eager "Yes!"
When you're getting it
on, silence isn't golden!

YOUR ULTIMATE ORGASM

Here's how to have that
mind-bending, unicorns-and-
rainbows feeling every time.

1. GIVE YOURSELF THE FINGER

If you need clitoral love during P-in-the-V, buzzing a fingertip vibe on your clitoris during doggie is a total treat.

2. GET IT IN BEFORE YOU START BARHOPPING

Not after. Alcohol makes you want to jump your bae's bones, but it produces vasocongestion, down-there swelling that keeps him from going deep, which can make it harder for you to finish. Tequila is a cruel mistress.

3. SEX SHOULDN'T FEEL LIKE *WINTER'S BONE*

Lube the eff up, please (both you and your partner, before and/or during the naughty). Almost 50 percent of women say lube makes it easier to orgasm. And forget the myth that it's just for older women. All the cool kids are doing it.

4. TELL HIM TO USE HIS FINGERS

He can use a finger (or two) while he uses his mouth on your Georgia O'Keeffe. Internal and external play is twice as nice for your orgasm chances.

5. KNOW YOUR LADY PARTS

Lest we (and he) forget, the clitoris extends down our labia in the shape of a wishbone. So he should lick or stroke the labia while down there. Wish-of-an-O, granted.

6. DO IT IN THE A.M.

Many women prefer getting it on in the morning. No beer slowing down the sparks, no calzone exacting revenge . . .

7. TRACK YOUR CRIMSON WAVE

Not only to save your undies, but also because on the thirteenth day of your cycle (right before you ovulate), your testosterone levels peak, resulting in a higher sex drive and bigger orgasm potential.

8. GET CLOSE

Most women need to feel close to someone to orgasm. You obvs don't need to get it on with a life partner to get off, but pick someone who's nice to you and you feel cares about you. Oh, and don't overlook this simple trick: Make eye contact. It feels so intimate that it can help you reach your peak.

ALL THE

Think of your orgasm less as a
with Kit Harington manning

CLITORAL
A go-to O for
many, thanks
to the clit's
8,000 sensory
nerve endings.

BLENDED
The swirl fro-yo
of orgasms,
stimulating your
clit and vagina
triggers more of
your brain,
resulting in more
pleasure.

SLEEPGASM
65 percent of
women climax
while asleep, due
to blood flow to
their Hope
Diamond. Good
night, indeed.

VAGINAL
The more rare
yet doable
O makes some
women report
full-body
tingles,
according to
research.

CERVICAL
Research
suggests the
vagus nerve
from the cervix
may be a
pathway to
(super-intense)
orgasms.

ORGASMS!

prix-fixe menu, more as an endless buffet
the build-your-own-omelet bar.

EARGASM

The vagus nerve
(the same one that
carries sensation
from the cervix)
also connects to
the ear. Wet Willy,
anyone?

BOOBGASM

Boobs = the
clitoris of your
chest. Nipple
stimulation can
activate the
same brain
region as clitoral
or vaginal love.

COREGASM

Get off the couch!
10 percent of
women report
feeling a deep
internal orgasm
while exercising.

ANALGASM

No butts about
it, the same
nether-region
nerve brings
pleasure to your
vagina, your
cervix, and your
bum.

THINKING OFF

The brain really
is a sex organ.
Some women
say they can O
just by *thinking*
about something
pleasurable.

←

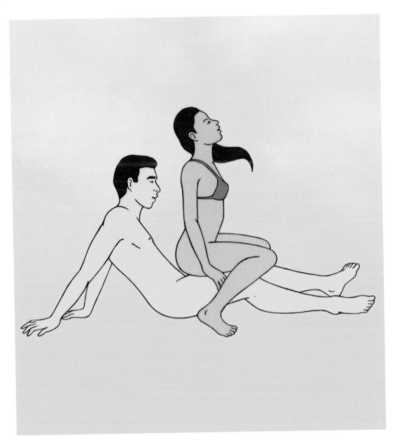

Twerk-Out Plan

Start with him sitting, legs straight out. Squat over him and move up and down, balancing backward if you need to. The low-level penetration stimulates the sensitive outside inches of your lady parts and the tip of his ween. Warning: Watching your booty bounce right in front of him might make his eyes bug out.

NEXT-LEVEL IT: **Transition onto your knees to get him deeper and continue to drop it like the temps in December.**

The Inner Circle

In-and-out can be kinda meh with a small member, so try a circular grinding motion instead. Get on your back, tuck a pillow under your butt, and open your legs wide. Have him enter you and grind against each other, rubbing your clit against his pubic bone in slow circles that turn into gotta-have-you faster ones.

MAKE IT HOTTER: **When he's about to lose it, place your feet on the bed and push down to create more tension for your grinding.**

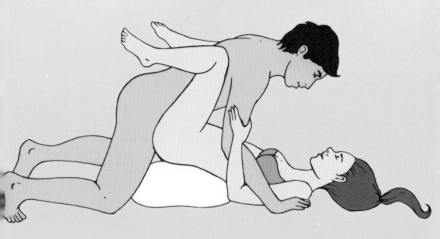

A gentle two-finger tapping motion against your G-spot will stimulate the area pre-deed. Try it yourself, or have your guy slip two fingers inside you and alternate taps with each fingertip.

Swirl Cone

We all scream for . . . this take on 69, which involves licking him like a soft-serve cone on a thousand-degree day. Start by swirling your tongue around the sensitive tip of his penis while your hips follow suit, moving in a circular motion over his mouth. (This means his tongue hits every spot of you.) See which one of you melts first.

SWITCH IT UP: **Instead of circular motions, try rocking your head side to side as you slide your mouth up and down.**

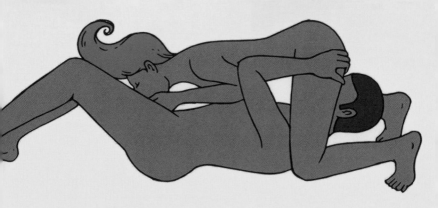

The Get-It Glide

Massage oil all over each other's chests, stomachs, and thighs. Then he'll enter you in missionary with your legs pressed tightly together, maximizing the slippery chest-to-chest contact while letting you control pressure on his peen. It's a hot mess (emphasis on *hot*), but totally worth it.

MAKE IT HOTTER: **Literally hotter. Instead of regular massage oil, try a candle that melts into massage oil. It's mood lighting and foreplay all in one!**

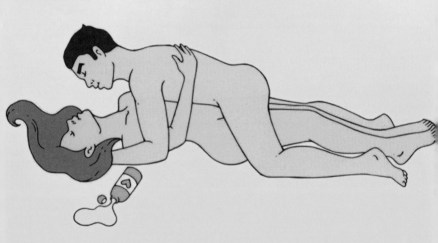

Have sex every day for a month. More frequent encounters rev your libido. Sex begets sex—you'll never want him more!

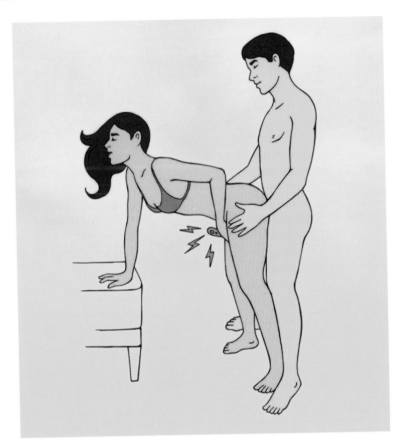

The Buzzy Bee

Stand by the edge of the bed, bending over with your hands on the mattress, as he enters you from behind. You get to be the Queen Bee here, using the vibe to buzz on your clit just the way you like it, while he gets deep penetration.

NEXT-LEVEL IT: **Let him be the worker bee. Hand him the vibe so he can have a turn to make you feel sweeter than honey.**

Side Bangs

Lie on your sides facing each other's crotches. Open your legs and go down on each other, just like a 69, but on your side. You can even rest your head on her inner thigh. Simultaneously getting each other off without the neck strain? Yes, please!

SWITCH IT UP: **Use a finger or two to massage each other's G-spots as your mouths work their magic.**

FOR GIRLS
WHO LOVE
GIRLS!

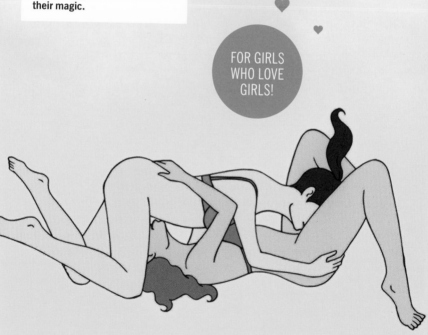

PART 3

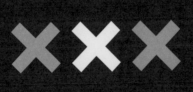

BURN THE SHEETS

IT DOESN'T GET HOTTER THAN THIS. YOU DON'T HAVE TO BE A CONTORTIONIST OR AN INDUSTRY PROFESSIONAL TO TRY THESE HIGH-LEVEL MOVES— BUT YOU DO HAVE TO BE READY FOR ADVENTURE (AND THE MOST MIND-BLOWING Os OF YOUR LIFE)!

Tantric Tub

While he reclines in a warm bath, climb on top so you're facing him. Once he's inside you, he'll sit up and you'll wrap your legs around each other, holding on to each other's knees. Sway back and forth to create internal friction. You'll feel like you're floating in more ways than one.

MAKE IT HOTTER: **Keep your sex going long past the pruney fingers stage with a silicone lube that will glide you along.**

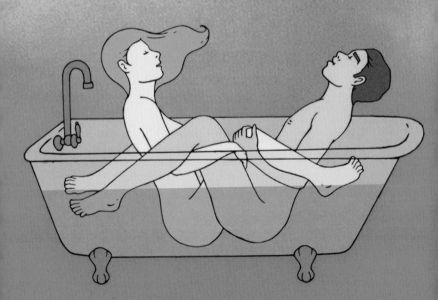

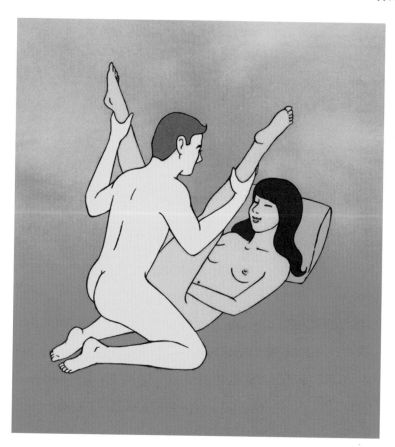

The Big V

While on your back, open your legs wide into the air (making a V shape) and let him grab your ankles while he thrusts. Not only is this move great for larger equipment, but you can also customize it as you go: He can move your ankles around and you have a hand free to rub your clit. Victory!

SWITCH IT UP: **Twist your hips to the right or left, leaving your legs wide open while he stays upright. With this twist, his hip will rub up against your clit as he moves in and out.**

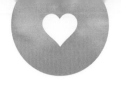

Make like a "Drunk in Love" Jay Z and Bey and just push your underwear aside to have sex. The immediacy of it is hot, like you just can't wait to have each other.

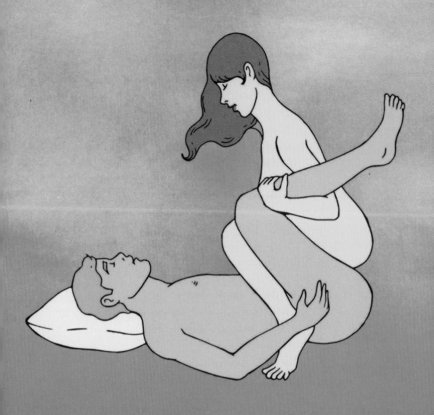

Slow-Motion Sensor

While lying on his back, he'll lift his knees to his chest. Straddle his hips and squat so your thighs hug the inside of his thighs. Lower yourself onto him slowly, taking him in, inch by inch, before getting your grind on. The slow-mo start will make every sensation feel more urgent.

MAKE IT HOTTER: **Before lowering yourself onto him, take your panties, bathrobe tie, or a pair of fuzzy handcuffs and tie his wrists to the bedposts so you're in total control of every movement.**

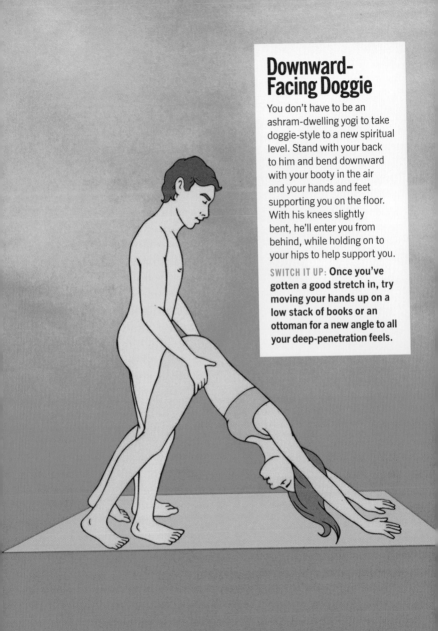

Downward-Facing Doggie

You don't have to be an ashram-dwelling yogi to take doggie-style to a new spiritual level. Stand with your back to him and bend downward with your booty in the air and your hands and feet supporting you on the floor. With his knees slightly bent, he'll enter you from behind, while holding on to your hips to help support you.

SWITCH IT UP: **Once you've gotten a good stretch in, try moving your hands up on a low stack of books or an ottoman for a new angle to all your deep-penetration feels.**

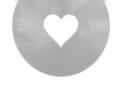

Sometimes we forget that men have super-sensitive nipples too. While your mouth is down below, reach up and trace sexy shapes— a heart, his name— all over his chest with your fingertips, making sure to hit his nipples.

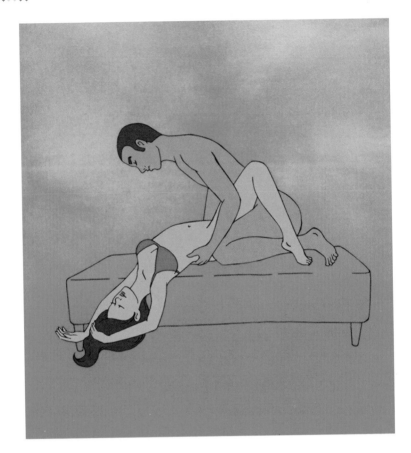

Daring Dangle

When you're in missionary, dangle yourself before him like the fine treat you are. Hang your head, shoulders, and arms off the bed while he's on top. You'll get a head rush. He'll get a sexy view.

NEXT-LEVEL IT: **Take it to the living room and drape yourself over the side of the living room couch. There's nothing hotter than wondering if a nosy neighbor might peep while you guys are getting it on.**

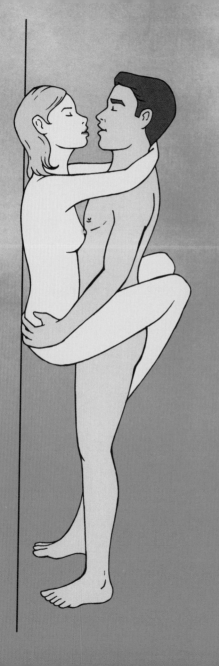

The Standing O

During a fierce make out where he's pushing you against a wall and grabbing your booty (natch), leap up into his arms. Lock your legs around his waist, hold onto his shoulders for leverage, and get busy. Sounds dramatic, but the upward angle gives your G-spot a clapping-emoji-worthy performance.

MAKE IT HOTTER: Kiss him everywhere . . . except for his mouth. Neck, jaw, cheeks, and forehead are all fair game in this super-close position.

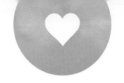

Scribble down a "menu" of the top three moves that drive you crazy, and invite him to do the same. Then swap lists, and take turns serving up the goods à la carte.

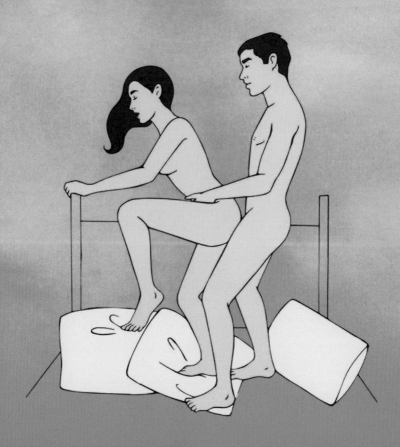

Merry Maid

The next time you're getting freaky on vacay, stand on the hotel-room bed pillows (not yours to wash!) and face the wall, grabbing onto a bedpost and propping a knee on the headboard. He'll enter you from behind, making every thrust feel super deep . . . and super dirty, especially if you're defiling a dainty bed-and-breakfast.

NEXT-LEVEL IT: **Role-play like you're the maid who's arrived for turndown service and he's all like, "Turn down for what?"**

The Frisky Fireworks

Lie on your back with your knees bent and your feet a foot or two apart. Then raise your hips up to the night sky and have him kneel between your legs and thrust away. The angle of your elevated hips will have his penis stroking the super-sensitive top of your vagina . . . and have you seeing fireworks.

SWITCH IT UP: **Open and shut your legs to feel yourself tighten around him. Add some well-timed Kegel squeezes and you'll both be ready to explode.**

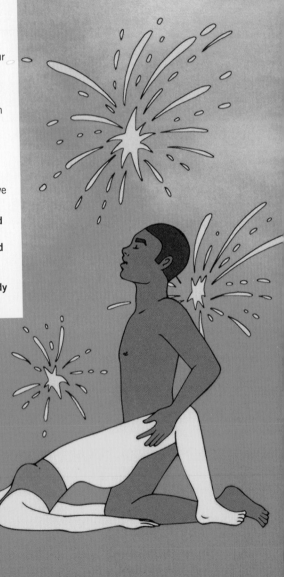

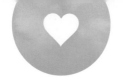

Get your dom on. Roll him onto his back and straddle him. Pin his hands down to his sides and clamp his legs shut with yours. Now run your lips and tongue all over his naked torso until he gets the shivers and begs you to go lower.

THREESOMES
Because the more the merrier, right?

Exactly How to
Have a Threesome

You might already have a perfect third
in mind (often a friend of yours who's game). If not,
go to a party or bar with your manfriend
and work your flirting magic on the ladies, as the
fire is often started with women. Or try
logging on to a hookup or dating site with threesome
categories. Whether you pick her up online
or in person, discuss the rules and what's on the
sexual menu before you get naked.
Also, use condoms.

How to Keep It Sexy and Fun

TALK ABOUT YOUR FEELINGS

Once you add a third person, there's often an emotional layer (jealousy, for example) that needs to be worked out. To keep the "Does he like her more than me?" voices at bay, acknowledge the insecurity and consciously decide to let it go so you can focus on the things you find sexy.

IMMERSE YOURSELF

The way she's moaning, the way he smells, the way their hands feel running up your body at the same time—focus on the good feelings to keep your mind from wandering to insecure places.

SIT BACK AND WATCH

Don't feel like everyone needs to be doing something at all times. Sometimes, the steamiest moments in a threesome can be watching two hot people enjoy each other.

Bounce House

While your guy is seated on the mattress with his legs crossed, hop onto his lap so you're straddling him in a kneeling position and holding on to his shoulders. Keep your bodies close and bounce gently into each other like you're the only two people home at the inflatable house.

NEXT-LEVEL IT:
Try it on an actual trampoline. So much bounce. So hot.

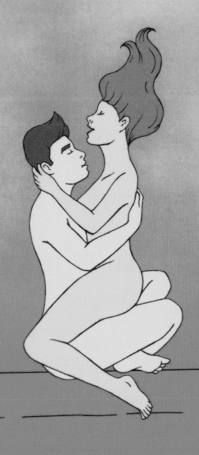

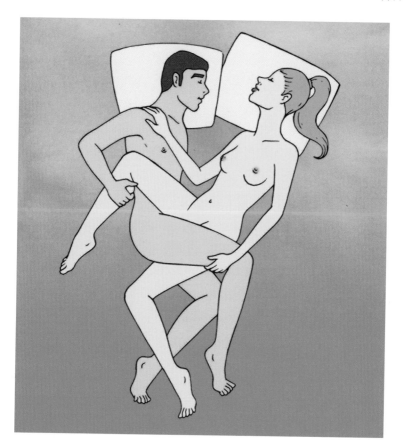

The Eternal O

Start in a spooning position, then lift your top leg back over his and turn your torso so you're on your back, facing him, with him still inside you. It's the perfect switch-up for practicing edging, aka getting completely turned on, then backing off right before you climax . . . so that you're always on the brink.

MAKE IT HOTTER: **Add a vibrating penis ring to the mix. If he wears it upside down, it'll vibe right up against your clit while you spoon.**

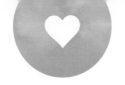

Use a vibe during oral sex. Place it against your cheek when you're down below so that he feels a rush of sensations all along his shaft. It is the beej equivalent of those Good Vibes Only posters.

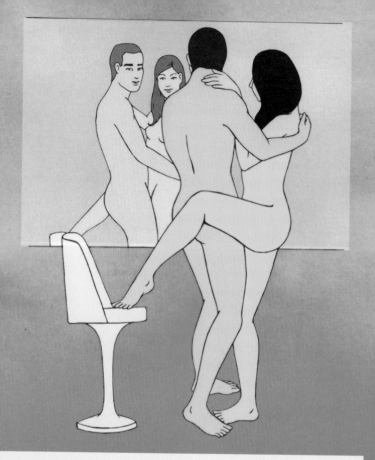

Be Your-Selfies

Drag a chair over to a full-length mirror and start making out, murmuring something like, "Look how hot we look." Tell him you want to watch while he slides inside you, and prop your leg up on the chair so you can see how completely sexy you look. Imagining that strangers are watching adds an extra layer of hotness to the deed.

NEXT-LEVEL IT: **Lower him slowly into the chair and hop on top with your booty facing the mirror . . . and take no offense when he stops kissing you to focus on your, um, rear-view mirror's reflection.**

Happy Crabs

With him in the crab-walk position (ya know, the one from gym class), stand, straddling his hips, and squat down to let him enter you. Lean back on your hands so you're now in a crab-walk position too but with him inside you. Once you lean back and start thrusting, all the G-spot stim will make you totally forget that you're working out those triceps too. Sexercise for the win!

SWITCH IT UP: **Take it to the floor. Doing the deed in any place other than a bed instantly makes it seem more taboo, aka hotter.**

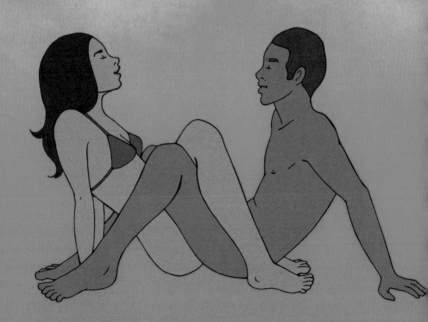

Bet that you can hold out from actual intercourse longer than he can. Then torment him with kisses on his neck and torso, softly stroke his inner thighs, and trail a lock of hair down his back to fire up his anticipation. Now it's his turn to make you wait!

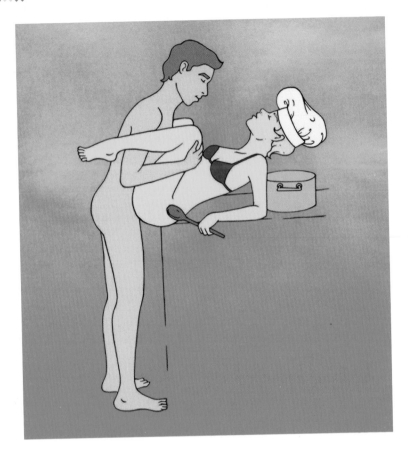

Yes, Chef

The next time you cook at home (or put takeout on plates, whatever), sit on the edge of your kitchen counter. Pull your knees up and arch your hips in a low bridge while he stands between your legs and brings you *his* delivery. Massaging your clit with his free hand is definitely on the menu.

NEXT-LEVEL IT: **Reach for the freezer, grab an ice cube, and run it along your body and his while you're doing the deed. It'll send chills (the good kind!) all over.**

Ab-Freaking Fab

Before he enters you in missionary, stack a couple of pillows under your butt, and when he leans forward to get busy, put your feet on his shoulders. It's a souped-up angle for your nerve-packed G-spot . . . and an ab workout because #Multitasking.

MAKE IT HOTTER: Use your hands to caress his face and neck, or twirl his hair around your fingertips, a major turn-on for some guys.

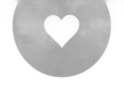

Make a playlist of sultry songs and set it to shuffle during sex. Change up your pace and mood to match each new tune. (Pro tip: Rihanna, *lots* of Rihanna.)

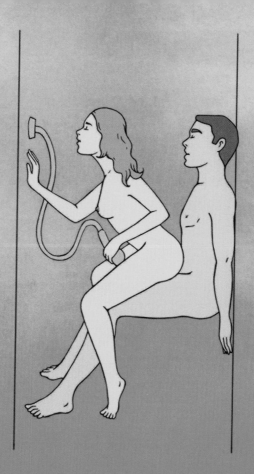

The Wet Down

After you've given each other soapy rubdowns (and rinse-downs), he'll squat while you reverse-straddle him, bracing yourself against the shower wall. Control the bounce with your legs while you give your clit attention with the detachable showerhead.

NEXT-LEVEL IT: **Speaking of shower "head" . . . start your shower session by kneeling down and treating him with your mouth.**

Take it outside.
Getting busy in a
public place is
a huge risk, thereby
doubling the
wattage of your hot
rendezvous.
Try wearing a skirt
with no undies,
and do it in a place
where you'll hear
someone coming, like
mid-stairwell.

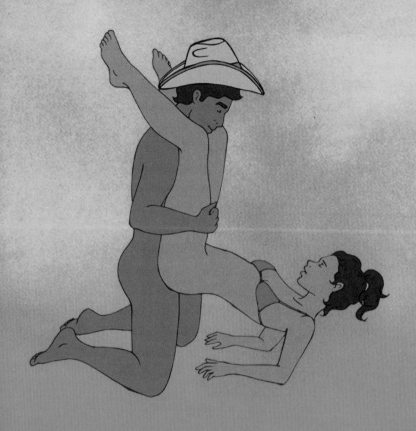

The Wild, Wild Best

Take him to the rodeo by leaning back on your elbows and hooking your legs over his shoulders (not as hard as it sounds, really). Then raise your butt slightly so you're hovering as he thrusts . . . um, howdy, partner. In the showdown of internal stimulation and easy clitoral access, it's a draw for which one will give you more pleasure.

SWITCH IT UP: Give your arms a rest and lean on your shoulders. Your bodies will be making more of an upside down V now, and the increased distance will make his in-and-out movements feel more intense.

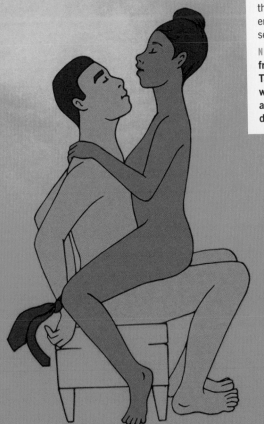

Frisky Business

Be the sexiest boss he's ever had: Bind his wrists with his silk tie, then sit your eager employee down on an ottoman or a chair and straddle him. Swivel your hips in figure-eights to vary the strokes for him and engage in a 360-degree love sesh for your vaginal wall.

NEXT-LEVEL IT: **Move the tie from his hands to his eyes. Taking away his visual cues will keep him guessing about what you're about to do to him next.**

While he's lying on his back in bed, lie perpendicular to his body with your head near his package. As you begin licking him, reach down with one hand and start rubbing yourself. Your positioning gives him an HD view of the whole program.

The Lusty Lift

You deserve a raise, sister! While you lie on your back, he'll face you, kneeling, and pull you up by your calves until your lower back is off the bed. He'll enter you in a downward angle that's a tight fit, thanks to your close-together thighs, and he gets to see the girls from a whole new angle.

MAKE IT HOTTER: Grab your breasts and push them together—did he just lose his mind? We thought so.

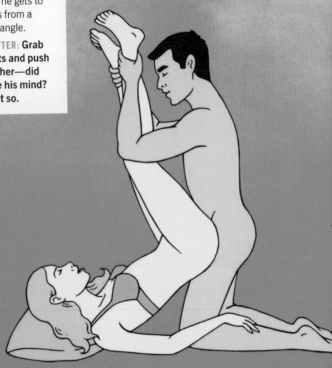

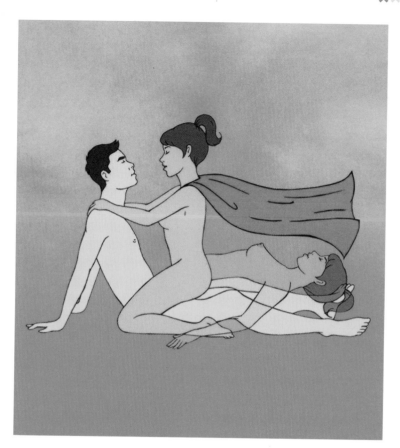

The Amazing Super-Girl

In missionary, hold his shoulders and wrap your legs around his waist. Use your superhero strength to swing upward, transitioning to girl-on-top. Pow! Bam! The quick change means he'll be hitting new spots inside you, and once you're on top, you can take full control and grind to your heart's delight.

NEXT-LEVEL IT: **Before you change positions, give his shoulders and neck a good rubdown. He'll be so Zen that he won't even see the switch-up coming.**

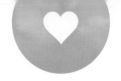

While standing with your back against his chest, ask him to reach around and touch you so that all you can see are his hands. Totally sexy.

Free-Floating Frolic

Find a penis-level table (the back of a sofa works too) and lie down on your stomach with your butt at the edge and your legs hanging over. Have him grab on to your hips, lifting your legs and holding them up. The penetration feels like you're floating on air—and hey, you kind of are, right?

MAKE IT HOTTER: Since you can't let your eyes tell him when you're about to lose it, use your indoor voice to whisper your thoughts, like, "You feel super deep inside me." He'll love the sexy feedback.

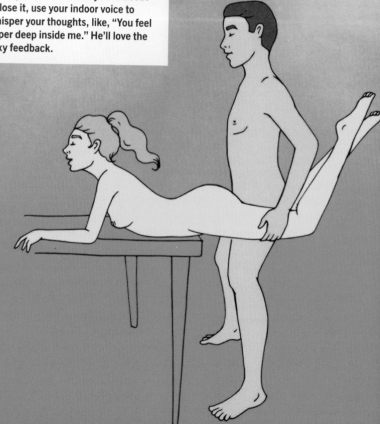

ROUGH SEX

Whether it's a little light spanking or full-on BDSM bonding, we say: May the force be with you.

In the era of equal rights and *Lean In,* it can be tricky for some women to admit that when the lights go off, they want to be dominated and pushed around a little, in the context of consensual play (which is, to be clear, what we're discussing here). But the truth is, many women do. Liking to be dominated doesn't mean you're damaged, it doesn't mean you're sexist, and it certainly doesn't mean you're okay with being bossed around in any other context. What makes rough sex sexy is the urgency factor—someone who wants you so badly, he can't stop himself from pinning you to the bed. Want to try it? Follow these steps.

START SMALL AND GO SLOWLY

Establish what's okay and what's not before even beginning, like saying force is cool, but name-calling isn't. Test out some light spanking or getting held down. Then if you're both comfortable, keep going.

RAMP UP THE INTENSITY

Try using restraints or slightly harder hitting. Always have a safe word at the ready (when you say "Bicycle," that means a hard stop), and make the dominant partner ask for what he or she wants, as in, "Can I spank you?" and then, "Yes, please spank me."

SWITCH IT UP

In terms of who's dominant, that is. That way you can both experience what it's like to be in control and what it's like to give it up.

As many as 57 percent of women are turned on by the idea of forceful sex, according to a University of North Texas study.

You don't have to choose between being a dom or a sub. Some people go both ways. They're called switches!

Submitting to someone else can be an aphrodisiac. The fact that you're willing to let go and indulge your darkest fantasies is pretty baller.

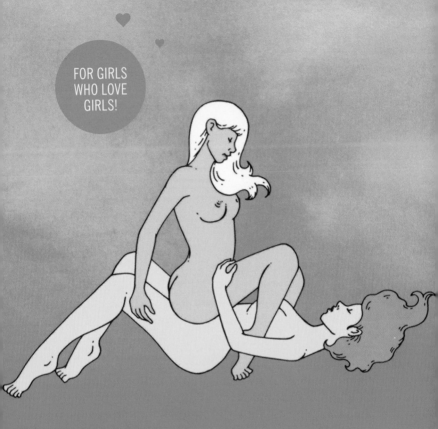

FOR GIRLS WHO LOVE GIRLS!

Sexy Sit-In

What do we want? Multiple Os! When do we want 'em? Now! Stand up for or, well, sit in for your right to set a steamy scene. While she's lying on her back, sit on her so your clits rub together. Rest your hands on her upper thighs for support while you grind. No protests here!

NEXT-LEVEL IT: Use your pointer finger to bring her nipples to attention—double the feels for her, super sexy visuals for you.

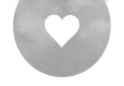

Take one or both of his testicles in your mouth. Hold there and swirl your tongue around or suck gently. They're a sensitive area, so light pressure is best (and most likely to drive him borderline insane).

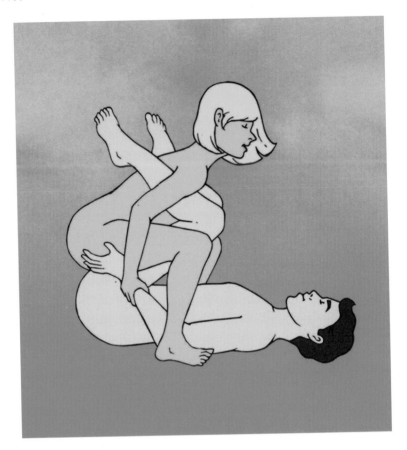

Vroom, Vroom

While he lies on his back with his knees toward his chest, face him and squat down, straddling his legs so your thighs are hugging his. Lower yourself onto his penis—the closer he draws his knees up to his chest, the better access you'll have—and bounce up and down. It's the ultimate rev-your-engines role reversal: He's curled up on his back, and you've mounted him like a Harley. Enjoy the ride.

NEXT-LEVEL IT: **Look into his eyes just as you're about to O. The intimacy of the moment will make him just die inside (the good way).**

The Work-It Wheelbarrow

While on your knees, cross your arms on the ground in front of you, using a pillow to cushion your elbows. Stick your butt in the air, and rest your head on your arms. He stands behind you and lifts your legs up by your ankles while you keep your knees bent. He enters you from behind, giving you both the benefits of doggie with the bonus of gravity on your side.

MAKE IT HOTTER: **Instead of straight-on in-and-out motions, having him swivel his hips from side to side while inside you will enhance your orgasm potential— the combo of a new angle and added movement excites hot spots you never knew you had.**

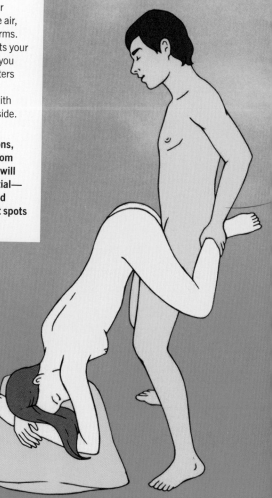

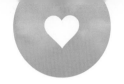

While he's still inside you catching his breath after an O, press your fingertips into his butt cheeks, kneading his skin. This wind-down move soothes him and reinforces your sexy bond.

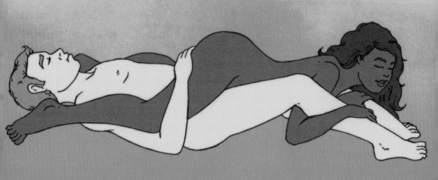

Slip 'n' Glide

Take control from the get-go and straddle him reverse-cowgirl style while he lies on his back. Then lower yourself onto him. Extend your legs back toward his shoulders, relaxing your torso forward onto the bed between his feet. Then slide forward and back, holding his ankles for added thrusting leverage. It's like having your own personal water slide ride . . . except way, way sexier.

NEXT-LEVEL IT: **Did someone say water slide? Lube up with a silicone formula that'll keep you slippery way past when the sun sets and the water park closes.**

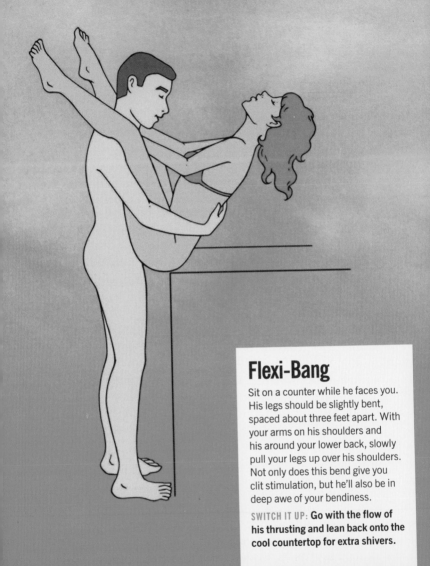

Flexi-Bang

Sit on a counter while he faces you. His legs should be slightly bent, spaced about three feet apart. With your arms on his shoulders and his around your lower back, slowly pull your legs up over his shoulders. Not only does this bend give you clit stimulation, but he'll also be in deep awe of your bendiness.

SWITCH IT UP: **Go with the flow of his thrusting and lean back onto the cool countertop for extra shivers.**

The area above his pelvic bone contains a cluster of sensitive nerve endings. Using a barely-there touch, trace across his lower tummy with your tongue—then blow his mind by blowing air along the same path.

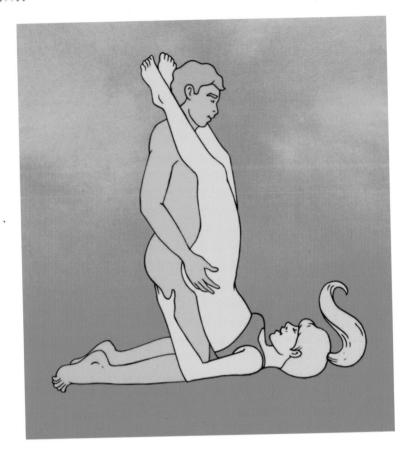

The A-Team

Lie flat on the ground, facing up. Lift your legs and butt way, way up in a shoulder stand. He kneels behind you, holding your hips while you drape your legs over his shoulders. Hold his thighs for leverage as he enters you. The blood rush to your thighs will intensify the sensations in the pelvic region, and he has perfect access to your happy place. Go team!

MAKE IT HOTTER: **If it's even possible to make this one steamier . . . run your finger up and down the back side of his thighs. Instant goosebumps.**

The Horny Helicopter

So he's entering you in traditional missionary when—whoa!—he does a 360-degree spin, all the while staying deep inside you. As he's rotating and thrusting, help guide him around you like a propeller. Plus, during his around-your-world revolution, you get to view every inch of his hot body.

NEXT-LEVEL IT: **You'll have direct access to his family jewels. Play with them gently as he thrusts.**

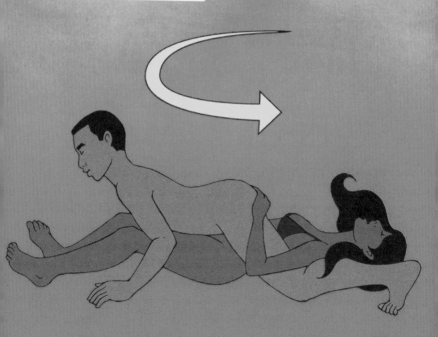

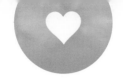

Take him to a random spot in your home where you've never done it before . . . and initiate a deep kiss and butt grab that lets him know how much you want him. Right here. Right now.

Gimme More

Take doggie-style to a whole new level of hotness with a vibrating butt plug. (Don't forget to lube up first!) He'll feel the vibes inside you, and as he thrusts, he'll push against the plug, making you feel doubly filled.

MAKE IT HOTTER: **Close your eyes so you can focus on every single sensation, especially if it's your first time testing the move out!**

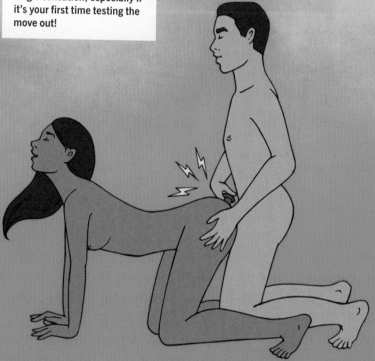

The Carnal Chair Pose

While he sits on a chair, straddle him and pull him inside you, then rock back and lean your arms on the ground. Then get ready for slow, gentle stimulation, deep penetration, and the general feeling of accomplishment from managing to get into a pretty hard-core pose.

SWITCH IT UP: Hand him a pebble vibe to press against your clit while you rock the night away.

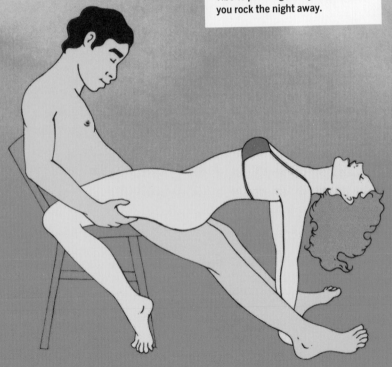

Try for a blended orgasm. Switch back and forth between touching your clitoris and stopping for him to thrust and hit your G-spot until you can't take it anymore. Then do both at the same time.

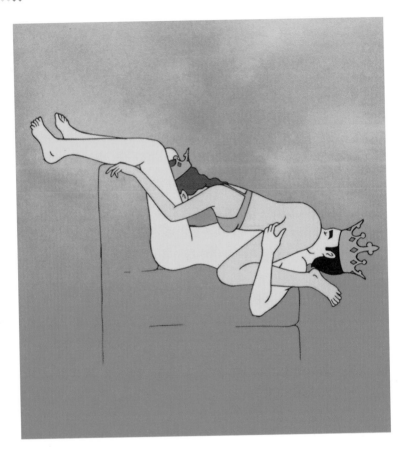

The Sofa King Amazing

We can think of one way to celebrate a successful trip to IKEA . . . . For this 69 upgrade, he lies on the sofa with his back and head on the seat and his legs draped over the back. Kneel over his face and bend down and go after it, as you both get your kicks.

NEXT-LEVEL IT: **Put your hands on his butt and massage his, um, cushions. His bum is a sexual pleasure point for him—who knew?**

Womanly Wrap

Lie on your back while she lies on top of you, also on her back. Reach around and place a vibrating wand on her clitoris in circular motions. The feeling of your breasts on her back is a major turn-on, while the wand works its orgasmic magic.

MAKE IT HOTTER: **Send shock waves to her brain by playing with one of her nipples with your free hand.**

FOR GIRLS WHO LOVE GIRLS!

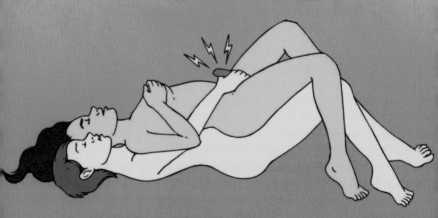

To keep him from blowing his fuse too early, try switching positions frequently. Spend just 30 seconds going down on him before moving on to another area, like his neck. Work that spot for a minute or so before moving back down.

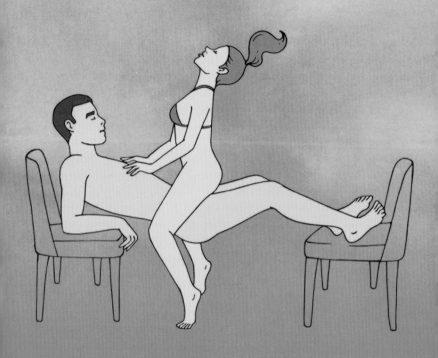

Bridge of Os

While he planks between two soft chairs, making himself into a literal man-bridge, ride him with your feet on the floor. You get to control the motion, and he gets an up-close view of your entire bod. We could get all funny here, but this one's intensity really will *bridge* you closer together.

MAKE IT HOTTER: How strong are his abs? Right before he's about to O, lift your feet off the ground to feel him pulse inside you.

KINK

Your guide to the power plays you never knew you had the (ben-wa) balls to try.

Master Being Master

SPANK YOU VERY MUCH

You're the HBIC, so put him to work. Guide him to gently rub one of your butt cheeks with his hand in long, slow strokes. Then tell him to increase the pressure before he plants a pat. The change of sensations will feel kinky without leaving your hot ass chapped. Feeling extra frisky? Upgrade to a cheeky paddle that leaves heart prints on your bum . . . and don't forget to punish him back.

LIGHT HIS FIRE

Turn up the flames with special candles that melt into warm body oils. Thrill him by dropping the warm, downstairs-friendly oil on his thigh. Then go to town massaging him right where he wants it. For extra spice, see if he's brave enough for a blindfold.

BABES IN TOYLAND

BDSM is known for its accessories, but if butt plugs and floggers freak you out, try storing a roll of bondage tape in your nightstand. When he least expects it, use the tear-and-wear restraints to tie his wrists to the bed or bind his hands behind his back. The magic tape sticks only to itself, not to skin, so it won't accidentally rip off his hair. And unlike handcuffs, there are no keys to lose in the abyss under your bed.

3 Secret Kink Props Hiding in Your House

HAIR ELASTIC
=
HANDCUFFS

Use it to bind his wrists.

HAIRBRUSH
=
PADDLE

Boar bristles feel naughty on a bare bum.

ELECTRIC TOOTHBRUSH
=
VIBRATOR

Hold the base against your clitoris during sex.

Show him how you touch yourself. (If you need a strong-ass vibrator, whip it out!) Guys love watching your one-woman show . . . and he'll be turned on enough to show you *his* solo moves. Take notes on what does it for him. Store away for later use.

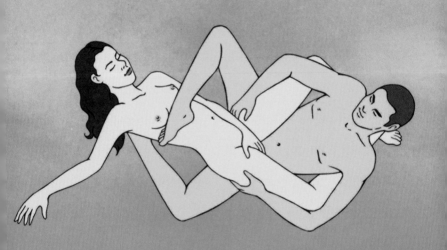

The Circle of Lust

While he lies on his back, straddle him and lower yourself onto him, but lean back, putting your arms between his legs. Then have him encircle your waist with his legs and thrust gently. This one is good for sensual G-spot tickling that goes slower than your parents' Wi-Fi. It's the kind that builds you up then brings your orgasm crashing down hard.

NEXT-LEVEL IT: **Guide one of his fingers to make windshield-wiper-like moves against your clit to take you over the edge.**

Cuddle. (It's not what you thought we'd say, right?) Couples who cuddle after sex (consider it after-play!) feel more satisfied with their sex lives and in turn, their relationship in general. And what's hotter than that?

INDEX